"An excellent introduction by two authors with deep knowledge of Jungian psychology who work in the fires of relationship. It suggests many useful approaches to therapists and couples who are struggling with understanding the complexity and challenges of 'living the couple.'"

Murray Stein, *Ph.D., author of* Jung's Map of the Soul

"This engaging book moves couples therapy into the depths of the soul. It links couples work into a more profound and resonant engagement with the depths of psyche and relationships."

Stanton Marlan, *Past President of the American Board and Academy of Psychoanalysis, Training and Supervising Analyst for the Inter-Regional Society of Jungian Analysts*

"A compassionate exploration of the unique challenges Jungian-oriented therapists face in working with the rich diversity of contemporary couples, in finding ways to support not only the individuation of each member of the couple but also to nurture the soul of the couple itself. The book's thoughtful review of core aspects of Jungian theory—typology, alchemy, the shadow— leads into its celebration of the archetypal basis of coupled life."

Christine Downing, *author of* Myths and Mysteries of Same-Sex Love

"As Jungian Psychology seeks to become a psychotherapy it reaches for some kind of authority in order to diagnose, interpret, and to treat. This move inevitably leads to various kinds of reduction, dissecting rather than obser- ving, the psyche. In *The Practice of Psychotherapy (CW 16)*, Jung confesses, 'If I wish to treat another individual psychologically at all, I must for better or worse give up all pretensions to superior knowledge, all authority and desire to influence' Jung embraces an approach to the psyche that honors its imaginal nature as a living participant in the work. In this book, Nelson and Delmedico work continually to remind us of the risk of this clinical reduction and insist that a Jungian approach to couple therapy rests upon this arche- typal foundation, the deepest strata of the unconscious. It welcomes images as alive and full of meaning."

Joseph Coppin, *PhD, Core Faculty Emeritus, Pacifica Graduate Institute, co-author* The Art of Inquiry: A Depth Psychological Perspective

"From the very beginning of this interesting and worthwhile book, readers are assured they are about to embark on something really meaty and something which is entirely lacking in the field. As Nelson and Delmedico make plain, trust in the slow, patient process of soulful couple therapy may seem as though the therapist is doing little during the hour, but nothing could be further from the truth. In a culture that prizes short-term therapy and measurable outcomes, listening for the murmurs of the soul asks more of us, not less."

Ruth Williams, *IAAP Training and Supervising Analyst, author of Jung*: The Basics and Exploring Spirituality from a Post-Jungian Perspective

"This book is an excellent resource for both therapists and lay people. It is solidly grounded in Jung's work and is written in a way that is creatively accessible and full of practical applications."

Allen Koehn, *D. Min., Former Director of the C.G. Jung Institute of Los Angeles, Professor Emeritus, Pacifica Graduate Institute*

"Elizabeth Nelson and Anthony Delmedico have provided a much-needed compendium of resources for therapists and teachers of couple therapy from a Jungian perspective. They have gathered the information, ideas, and perspectives informed by the depth psychology of Carl Jung and those who practice Jungian psychology so that readers don't have to search for diverse information about complexes, archetypes, typology, and unconscious dynamics in couple relating. If you practice, teach or supervise Jungian psychotherapy for couples, this book should be at your side because it is precise and comprehensive."

Polly Young-Eisendrath, *PhD, Jungian Analyst, author of* Love Between Equals: Relationship as a Spiritual Path and Hags & Heroes: A Feminist Approach to Jungian Psychotherapy with Couples

The Art of Jungian Couples Therapy

Within this accessible volume, Nelson and Delmedico apply a Jungian approach to provide fresh ways of thinking about couples therapy, and the profound unconscious forces at play when couples create a life together.

The Art of Jungian Couples Therapy offers new perspectives into thinking about what is happening in the consulting room, which the authors re-imagine as a sacred space or "temenos" guiding partners toward psychological wholeness, or what Jung termed the *Self*. The book offers welcome insights into how therapists can work with the complex and often intense energies that arise when two people cross the threshold of the clinical space. As "art" in the title suggests, it draws the therapist's attention to the souls of the partners and the soul of the relationship itself.

Firmly grounded in Jungian thought yet intimate, approachable, and up to date, the book will be an indispensable guide for professional marriage and family therapists, psychoanalysts from both Jungian and Freudian schools, counseling psychologists, and licensed social workers who already practice couples therapy or have considered working with couples.

Elizabeth Éowyn Nelson, PhD, Jungian scholar and international speaker, has taught at Pacifica Graduate Institute since 2003. She has published two books as well as several academic papers and individual chapters on diverse subjects including dream, feminism, film, mythology, technology, and research. She is on the board of the Jungian Society for Scholarly Studies and served as General Editor of the peer-reviewed *Journal of Jungian Scholarly Studies* for five years.

Anthony Delmedico, PhD, LMFT is a depth psychotherapist and AAMFT-Approved Supervisor in private practice in Raleigh, North Carolina. He has written about the depths of relationship, fatherhood, divorce, and sexual abuse.

The Art of Jungian Couples Therapy

An Introduction

Elizabeth Éowyn Nelson and Anthony Delmedico

Routledge
Taylor & Francis Group

LONDON AND NEW YORK

Designed cover image: Cover image by Lucy Stefani Nally. Used with permission.

First published 2026
by Routledge
4 Park Square, Milton Park, Abingdon, Oxon OX14 4RN

and by Routledge
605 Third Avenue, New York, NY 10158

Routledge is an imprint of the Taylor & Francis Group, an informa business

British Library Cataloguing-in-Publication Data
A catalogue record for this book is available from the British Library

ISBN: 978-1-032-68799-5 (hbk)
ISBN: 978-1-032-68798-8 (pbk)
ISBN: 978-1-032-68800-8 (ebk)

DOI: 10.4324/9781032688008

Typeset in Times New Roman
by Taylor & Francis Books

Contents

Illustrations

Figures

Tables

Excursions

Acknowledgements

Thanking everyone who made this book possible is impossible. Numberless teachers, mentors, students, colleagues, clients, and friends shape an author's ideas—not to mention the ancestors whose living ideas inform the work. To all of these, we owe immense gratitude. The soul of the book has been a steady companion, inspiration, and taskmaster.

Four dedicated Jungian scholar-clinicians granted us their time and attention to review the work in its entirety, and we thank them for their generosity: Luke Hockley, Allen Koehn, Murray Stein, and Ruth Williams.

Another group of people, experts in their subject matter, agreed to review individual chapters for us. We are deeply grateful to each of them: Stanton Marlan for his expert tending of the couples retort in the alchemy chapter; Joseph Coppin for his soulful reflections on the Introduction, Chapter 3 and Chapter 8; John Beebe for his subtle and keen insights in his review of the typology chapter; Patricia Berry, one of the founders of archetypal psychology, for her review of the archetypal chapter; and Christine Downing and Doug Thomas for their perceptive insights on the diversity chapter.

We also wish to thank Pacifica Graduate Institute's research librarians Mark Kelly and Richard Buchen for their invaluable help finding Jungian needles in haystacks far and wide.

Anthony would like to thank Annie Delmedico for her editing of an early chapter draft which helped inspire and fuel the work. Thank you, Elizabeth, co-writer, for your willingness to hang in there during our underworld journey together. Alchemy, indeed! Thank you, Hope Panara, for unwavering support and belief. A greater gift may not be found.

Elizabeth is grateful to Geoff—beloved husband, dear friend, fellow writer, and cat dad extraordinaire—for everything she has learned about marriage and about herself in the last two decades. Dear friends, keen to hear reports from the front lines of the writing life, were staunch allies; she is especially thankful for the subtle editing eye of her creative writing partner, Shaler McClure Wright. To my graduate students, from whom I continue to learn so much: you bring me joy. And finally, a wholehearted thank you to Tony. You have been a dear co-author who, even in the most challenging moments, made me laugh.

A Prologue In the Form of Epigraphs

The more one sees of human fate and the more one examines its secret springs of action, the more one is impressed by the strength of unconscious motives and by the limitations of free choice. The doctor knows—or at least he should know—that he did not choose this career by chance.[1]

C. G. Jung

We fall in and out of love or are carried and redeemed, or cursed, through its working, but that which love works upon is not love but soul.[2]

James Hillman

Go deeper than love, for the soul has great depths.[3]

D.H. Lawrence

The life-long dialectical encounter between two partners ... can be understood as a special path for discovering the soul, as a special form of individuation.[4]

Adolph Guggenbuhl-Craig

[1] Jung, C. G. (1954). The psychology of the transference. *The practice of psychotherapy, Collected Works, Vol. 16*, 2nd Edition Revised and Augmented. Princeton University Press. Used with permission conveyed through Copyright Clearance Center, Inc.

[2] Hillman, J. (1985). *Anima:An anatomy of a personified notion*. Spring Publications. Used with permission.

[3] *The Cambridge edition of the works of D.H. Lawrence: Poems, Volume 1* (2013) © Cambridge University Press 2013. Reproduced by permission of Paper Lion Ltd, The Estate of Frieda Lawrence Ravagli and Cambridge University Press.

[4] Guggenbuhl-Craig, A. (1977). *Marriage dead or alive* (M. Stein, Trans.). Spring Publications. Used with permission.

The fact that we cannot really know the soul and spirit of another person is exactly what love is about, for love means to establish an intimate relationship with the not-known.[5]

Robert Sardello & Robert Simmons

The soul of marriage ... is created by small acts, small words, and small, every day interactions.[6]

Thomas Moore

Marriage—I've tried it. Indeed I've been married more years of my life than I've been single, and those were the main mature conscious years. But I haven't a clue what makes it work and not work, discern which is which, or whether that word "work" is applicable at all.[7]

James Hillman

We two form a multitude.[8]

Ovid

Known to the world as "the perfect couple," basking in how they look to others, they wither behind their perfect masks.[9]

Marion Woodman

From the place where we are right
flowers will never grow
in the spring.[10]

Yehuda Amichai

beginning glistens
on all the breaking places of our failure.[11]

Rainer Maria Rilke

5   Sardello, R. (2008). *Love and the soul.* Goldenstone Press, Heaven & Earth Publishing, and North Atlantic Books. Used with permission.
6   From *Soul mates* by Thomas Moore. Copyright 1994 by Thomas Moore. Used by permission of HarperCollins Publishers.
7   Hillman, J. (1996). Marriage, intimacy, freedom. *Spring*, 60, 1–11. Used with permission. Spring Publications.
8   Behnam, W. G. (1924). *Benham's Book of quotations, proverbs, and household words.* Ward, Lock & Company, Limited. Public Domain.
9   Woodman, M. (1985). *The pregnant virgin.* Inner City Books. Used with permission.
10 Amichai, Y. (1986). From the place where we are right. *The selected poetry of Yehuda Amichai.* University of California Press. Used with permission.
11 Rilke, R. M. (1975). *Rilke on love and other difficulties* (J. I. L. Mood, Trans.). W. W. Norton & Company. Used with permission.

Introduction

When most people think of psychotherapy, they imagine one therapist working with one patient. Many therapists, however, find it deeply gratifying to work with couples in addition to working with individuals. This book is dedicated to the particularities and challenges of couples therapy. It is intended both for experienced therapists seeking ways to deepen their approach and for newer clinical interns who are beginning to imagine how to hold the couple and themselves in the therapeutic container. We imagine that *The Art of Jungian Couples Therapy* will also appeal to troubled partners in search of new ways to understand the mysteries of their relationship, including its frustrations, in the overall context of the meaning and purpose of their lives.

The serious wounds that afflict couples, like the wounds that bring individuals to therapy, are often years in the making, and the need for care is urgent. Working with wounded (and wounding) partners in such a state—sitting knee-to-knee with them and listening to their stories of heartbreak—is but one reason couples therapy is so difficult. Another equally important reason is something that forced itself on Carl Jung's attention throughout his long years of analytical work and personal experience: the mysteries of love surpass *rational* understanding. Eros, once imagined as a god, simply cannot be comprehended or explained away since his "range of activity extends from the endless spaces of the heavens to the dark abysses of hell."[1] Couples seeking therapy know this. They have been there. They, too, are bewildered; not by the heights of love, but by its more torturous depths, which no one can prepare for.

When couples cross the threshold into clinical space, four souls will need attention: the soul of each partner, the soul of the therapist, and the soul of the relationship itself, because the relationship, too, is alive; it, too, evolves as a couple grows together and grows apart in large ways and small. Little wonder that couples therapists seeking ways around and through complex relational dynamics are eager for simple, reliable techniques and new tools to rescue suffering couples and ease the burden of the work.

Though not all psychotherapists choose to work with couples, it is fair to say that all therapists work with the wounds of love. The echo, image, or ghost of an absent partner is present in the clinical space, whether overtly

DOI: 10.4324/9781032688008-1

recognized or not. Sitting with troubled patients who are suffering love's wounds is a sacred endeavor. The therapist's office, dedicated to the work, also becomes a sacred place for listening to souls *in extremis*.

Reimagining therapy as sacred work is a core aspect of a Jungian approach, returning it "to the province of spiritual practice, as was the case in antiquity,"[2] says Lionel Corbett. The therapist hopes to awaken a couple's longing for something ineffable and unnamable, perhaps something they once felt with each other but now have lost. Such an orientation deepens and enriches the clinical space, transforming therapy into an art that entails "the conscious use of skill and creative imagination."[3] In time, a couple may come to experience encounters with mystery and persistent questions of meaning as psychologically valuable.

The emphasis on the spiritual dimension of human life is, indeed, Jung's most important legacy.[4] Two brilliant analysts who worked closely with Jung assert this point. Aniela Jaffé, Jung's colleague and editor of his memoir, says simply, "life, for Jung, is lived only when it is 'a touchstone for the truth of the spirit.'"[5] Marie-Louise von Franz, another revered colleague, speaks of Jung's emphasis on "inner experience which is as old as mankind ... when something alien and unknown overwhelms us from within, when the workings of inner forces suddenly changes our lives."[6] For millennia, the eruption of such inner experiences has been explained as the incursion of the sacred into ordinary life. These experiences cannot be measured, duplicated, or predicted. They are utterly unique. At the same time, the phenomenon of spiritual experience—a sense of the sacred shared across cultures and throughout time—is evident in cosmologies from every part of the globe, which offered Jung abundant historical evidence to assert the central importance of spirituality to human psychology.

The ubiquity of spiritual experience has led Jungians to speak of a religious instinct, a collective human capacity expressed universally in myth, dream, and ritual. The collective unconscious, also known as the objective psyche, is like a compendium of ancestral memories, a great, cumulative encyclopedia of archetypal patterns, figures, and motifs. We say more about the religious instinct, archetypes, and the collective unconscious throughout the book. For now, it is enough to say that the source of Jungian insight into couples' lives is rooted in something far deeper and more timeless than many current treatment approaches allow and account for.

Jung found that "spiritual longings, beliefs and experiences stemmed from the psyche's intrinsic striving toward wholeness, which required that the individual move beyond, and expand, their everyday view of themselves."[7] A Jungian approach, in contrast to other kinds of couples therapy, is dedicated to wholeness. It encourages the expansion of the partners' everyday view of themselves individually, as well as their view of the relationship, by opening themselves to the contents bubbling up from the unconscious. It goes one step further, imagining the dynamic unconscious as an active presence in the relationship. From a Jungian perspective, relationship is a spiritual experience in which two souls are dancing together, each trying to work out the rhythms of the partnership, sometimes with a modicum of grace and sometimes without it. Reimagining couples therapy as care of two dancing souls caught in their conflicts alters many things, perhaps especially how therapists and partners regard suffering. When they can regard suffering as meaningful and necessary, they honor the soul and demonstrate faith in the slow, mysterious, circular processes of psychological growth.

Transformation of the soul of the relationship, as well as the soul of each partner, requires deepening down into the dark and fertile soil of the unconscious. Faith in this process is radically countercultural because it is slow, because it is mysterious and circular, and ultimately because it challenges the Western fantasy of tidy interventions and evidence-based results. As Thomas Moore says, care of the soul "isn't about curing, fixing, changing, adjusting" or restoring the partners or the relationship to so-called health so that they can enjoy a trouble-free future, guided by "some idea of perfection or even improvement."[8] Rather, therapy as a spiritual practice on behalf of soul "remains patiently in the present, close to life as it presents itself day by day."[9]

Trust in the process can sometimes make it appear as though the therapist is doing little during the clinical hour, but nothing could be further from the truth. In a culture that prizes short-term therapy and measurable outcomes, listening for the murmurs of the soul asks more of us, therapists and couples alike, not less.

Four Philosophical Assumptions and a Quintessence

Four essential assumptions underlie this book's approach. First, as James Hillman says, it is impossible to know ourselves by ourselves because "the soul needs intimate connection, not only to individuate but simply to live."[10] Moore says something similar when he describes love as an "an event of the soul"[11] that broadens our vision of ourselves, of our partners, and of the world.

Next, for many people, relationships are a necessary part of the individuation journey. Profound and durable commitments frequently touch and transform partners in ways that are impossible without it. When two people create a life together that extends beyond the first honeymoon period, they almost inevitably experience not only the expansive heavens but also as the dark abysses of hell with each other.

Third, relationships are sacred, living mysteries in which partners dance along the edge between the known and the unknown. The mysterious depths of relationship include each partner's personal and cultural shadow, all that remains unspoken and possibly unconscious between them. Indeed, it may be that the story that has not yet been told has brought them to the threshold of therapy.

Finally, some couples seek (or are reluctantly brought into) what Jung calls a *psychological marriage*, one that is dedicated to the journey toward wholeness for both partners and the relationship. In psychological relationships, couples inevitably experience discomfort and conflict since "there is no birth of consciousness without pain."[12] They come to recognize conflict as an integral aspect of the relationship's growth because the relationship, too, is a living psychological process with its own soul working out its own destiny.

What unites these four philosophical assumptions is the quintessence of *soul*. This book follows a long philosophical tradition in the West, including such thinkers as Heraclitus, Plato, and Marsilio Ficino, to make care of the soul its central concern.[13] Equally important, *The Art of Jungian Couples Therapy* takes seriously Jung's lament that psyche was rarely spoken with, always spoken about, because "the soul was never able to get a word in."[14] A Jungian approach encourages listening to each partner's psyche and keeping those needs close. Of any event, thought, or feeling between the partners, therapists might ask: *How is this the soul speaking?* As Moore says, relationships are the place where soul works out its destiny, a most intimate space to wonder about the soul's own purposes.[15] Re-valuing soul in couples therapy is not necessarily a move against ego, but it does de-center ego concerns. It questions the value of heroic, ego-based striving, which may, for the sake of the illusion of a perfect coupled life, lead to the repression of necessary conflicts and ignore the need of the soul to dwell in the vales of difficulty.

The soul of the relationship, where suffering and symptom intersect, is ignored by much of the therapeutic profession that purportedly has the expertise to deal with it. Valuing love's difficulties is not easy. Not for the partners. Not for the therapist. For therapists, the archetypal energies of hero or savior are acutely activated and they manifest in unrelenting conscious and unconscious pressures to save relationships. Couples often arrive to therapy in regressed states and desperate enough to reveal their depths to strangers.[16] Because relationships have their own fates (a bitter truth for untempered egos to accept and remember), the only authentic move for therapists is to help couples enter the mystery of what is occurring between them and inside them. That is precisely where Jung's psychology excels, and it is what we hope this book will illuminate. We want to usher readers further into the mystery of relationship—the *eros* of it—while hopefully providing enough *logos* to get across the threshold.

The poet Rainer Maria Rilke speaks of marriage as a "great, demanding claim" that calls a person to "vast distances ... the ultimate, perhaps that for which human lives are as yet barely large enough."[17] This is true for some couples but not for all. Some partners remain happily unconscious and content in what Jung called *conventional marriages*.[18] These are not the couples who typically come for therapy. The troubled couples who do show up are usually in relationships that no longer allow them to remain unconscious together. Instead, the relationship is now demanding more consciousness and with this demand there comes a painful loss of innocence. The loss of the ideal relationship (and partner) that each person had been dreaming into puts tremendous psychological pressure on the individuals and on the relationship itself. Working with couples also lays a great, demanding claim on therapists, confronting them with profound questions, including those about their own attempts at lifelong commitment.

Psychotherapy is fundamentally, irreducibly relational. This means the therapist's soul and their wounds are also in the work, whether they are conscious of them or not. It cannot be otherwise. Therapists sometimes forget that they, too, are also real, living, hurting, hurtful, limited and vulnerable human beings, often working through their own relational needs and problems. They believe instead that they have acquired some superhuman ability to remain detached, bracketing out their own soul and their own humanity from the therapeutic equation. Freud's early recommendation was to practice listening with an "evenly-suspended attention."[19] It is a laudable goal, but reality is that attention wanders, snags, and is drawn into the couple's drama. Therapists simply cannot remain untouched by the stories they hear day in and day out.

Considering the depth and intensity of love's wounds, the practice of couples therapy requires immense courage. And because of the utter uniqueness of each therapist, each partner, and each relationship, there is simply no one right way to do it. The question motivating this book is: *What can a Jungian approach to working with couples offer the therapist?* Our book does not ask therapists to dispense with their acquired knowledge, skill, and expertise. Rather, the aim is to explore new ways of being with couples that expand and deepen more familiar techniques. Jung asserts it is the whole person of the therapist that matters. "Every psychotherapist not only has his own method— he himself is that method ... The great healing factor in psychotherapy is the doctor's personality."[20]

Jung's personality shaped not only his analytic practice, but it also drove his appetite for the widest possible range of knowledge. He was an edge-dweller, with one foot in the personal world of his patients' stories and one foot in the timeless world of myth, archetypal figures, situations, and themes, the objective psyche.[21] An embodied Jungian couples therapy begins in this double stance, one foot grounded in present-day reality, attuned to the partners' personal stories, the other foot planted in the transpersonal world of the unconscious. Edge-dwelling accounts for the wholly different feel of Jungian therapy since, as Jung admits, there is an "extraordinary timeless quality of the unconscious: everything has already happened and is yet unhappened, is already dead and yet unborn."[22] Therapists curious about the unconscious can begin by exploring the intriguing motifs and figures that show up weekly in the clinical setting, regarding them as timeless qualities expressing the never-ending intricacies of coupled life.

Patterns of thought, belief, and behavior recur across multiple domains: individual, familial, communal, cultural, and mythic.[23] Recognizing these

recurring relational patterns as *archetypal*—that is, valuable and meaningful—is a skill therapists develop throughout their professional lives. The
patterns come to be seen not just as repetitive, but as universal and even
necessary. Approaching archetypal material with a sense of wonder usually
leads the curious investigator of the unconscious to the pattern's deeper roots.
Over time, therapists will recognize similar themes and patterns in other cultures and other storytelling traditions. Sharing these universal similarities
during the clinical hour can expand a couple's perspective, adding richness
and meaning to their struggle and help them to transform their story into *the*
story. Ultimately, knowledge of archetypal patterns can create a kind of home
for partners' emotional and spiritual lives, giving them a sense of belonging.

The Map is not the Territory

Throughout Jung's analytic career with individual patients, he also worked
with countless couples.[24] He left suggestions about the analytic process and a
generative approach but no maps or instructions. Jung's metapsychology
picks up where much of contemporary psychotherapy training leaves off. This
is precisely where his work begins to sparkle, shine, and illuminate—without
offering reductive prescriptions for fixing or saving. It situates itself at that
place that Dante speaks of so hauntingly:

> In the middle of the journey of our life, I came to myself, in a dark wood,
> where the direct way was lost. It is a hard thing to speak of, how wild,
> harsh and impenetrable that wood was, so that thinking of it recreates the
> fear. It is scarcely less bitter than death.[25]

Jung's psychology focuses on the unconscious, the place from which unseen
and often overwhelming forces arise. For therapists, nowhere are those invisible forces more on display than in working with couples. Therapists usually
get the *live feed* with couples—tensions on full, dramatic display in the heat of
the moment—in sharp contrast to still painful but perhaps less intense energies more often present in individual therapy. Working so intensely with a
couple's individual and shared complexes often activates the therapist's own
complexes. The head of the Medusa is everywhere; if therapists look at her
face directly, she will turn them to stone. In such treacherous environments,
some therapists grasp at technique to survive the clinical encounter. They may
try to break relational dynamics into stages, hand out worksheets, prescribe
date nights, and so on—all well-meaning attempts to quell the intense energies rising from the unconscious.

The Art of Jungian Couples Therapy honors the heart-hewn and fire-tem-
pered psychologies unique to each Jungian analyst, Jungian-informed therapist, and Jungian scholar. It does not offer a systematized Jungian approach
to couples therapy but instead establishes that same respect for the Jungian-

informed couples therapist. All therapists wander the path of individuation, whether they are aware of it or not, simply because the work demands it. A Jungian approach provides a supportive framework for this wandering, personally and professionally. It asks therapists to re-value the Self, which includes re-valuing their own thinking, feeling, sensing, and intuition in the consulting room. It also asks therapists to respect and re-value their own embodied sense of what is going on below the stormy surface of troubled clinical waters. In the end, all profound relationships—including the therapist's commitment to their art, to the couples they work with, and to their own psyche—provide an incomparable opportunity to sojourn with the hidden and often unvoiced depths of human suffering. And when couples therapists find themselves wholly lost and in the dark, personally or in the consulting room, we hope Jung's work will light the way.

Organization and Style

Many excellent primers on Jungian theory already exist, including works by Edward Edinger, Aniela Jaffé, Murray Stein, Anthony Storr, David Tacey, Marie-Louise von Franz, Ann Yeoman and Kevin Lu, Polly Young-Eisendrath and Terence Dawson.[26] *The Art of Jungian Couples Therapy* does not replace them: it discusses only core Jungian concepts that influence coupled life and couples therapy. These include Jung's notions of the collective unconscious, individuation, complexes, shadow, anima/animus, typology, alchemy, archetypal figures, soul, and the psyche. Establishing their meaning in the context of couples therapy introduces readers to a language that fosters new ways of thinking, imagining, and being with troubled couples that complement current mainstream approaches.

Although the book necessarily introduces some of Jung's terminology, we have tried to avoid specialized jargon wherever possible. We remained close to the roots and trunk of the Jungian tree, ever aware of the dense and far-reaching breadth of Jung's writing and the hundreds of Jungian authors who have extended his thinking. Aiming at brevity and introductory clarity has led to some notable over-simplifications and painful editorial choices. For example, those familiar with Jung's psychology will notice some glaring omissions such as working with dreams,[27] imaginal dialogues,[28] the transcendent function,[29] and sand play.[30] All are useful in working with couples, and we encourage curious readers to explore the topics independently.

Because the concepts described in this book are alive in the psyche, we depart from the norm and use present tense verbs to reflect this liveliness, e.g., "Jung said ..." becomes "Jung says ...". This choice honors the timelessness of soul and psyche, even if it irritates the ego. We use gender-neutral pronouns wherever possible without altering the original (often masculine) pronouns in direct quotes. Some quotes reference marriage but the concepts apply in any emotionally committed relationship.

As the title intimates, *The Art of Jungian Couples Therapy* does not offer simple techniques or new solutions. Clinical vignettes are rarely included since case material can be a step on the path toward a reductive manualized approach. Departing from the usual and customary *what to do*, readers are invited to step more fully into *how to be*. Although therapy with individuals is alive, emergent, and unfolds uniquely moment by moment, working with couples adds layers of complexity and nuance. Readers will also notice occasional excursions throughout *The Art of Jungian Couples Therapy*, detours that temporarily step away from the narrative flow in order to highlight a theme or concept in a novel way.

We hope you will consider the themes amplified in this book on their own merit and think about their personal and professional implications. Perhaps, above all, we hope you will allow associations to the ideas and images presented in *The Art of Jungian Couples Therapy* to arise naturally in your own mind, heart, and soul.

Bibliographic Note

We have favored primary sources and limited the number of in-text references to make the book easier to read while providing enough documentation for readers to locate source material. We also simplified the reference section at the end of each chapter by omitting many subtitles. The abbreviation *CW* denotes Jung's *Collected Works*; for example, *CW* 6 is Jung's *Collected Works*, Volume 6, citing the original publication date of an essay or the volume publication date when referring to the entire work. Because Jung's *Collected Works* have appeared in a variety of versions and editions, when citing his work, we use paragraph numbers (para.) instead of page numbers. Jung's *Collected Works* were edited by Herbert Read, Michael Fordham, Gerhard Adler, and William McGuire, translated from German by R. F. C. Hull, and are published by Princeton University Press in the United States and Routledge in England. *SE* is used to denote Freud's *Standard Edition* (e.g., *SE* XXI is Volume 21 in the *Standard Edition of the Complete Psychological Works of Sigmund Freud*), citing the original publication date of the essay. The *Standard Edition* is edited and translated by James Strachey and published by Hogarth Press in London.

Notes

1 Jung 1989 [1961], p. 412.
2 Corbett 1996, p. 5.
3 *Merriam-Webster* n.d., art.
4 To gain some appreciation for the public's idea of Jungian psychology, consider, for example, a 2024 Google search that posed the question, "What is Carl Jung's most famous idea?" The first answer was "his recognition of the psychological value of spiritual experience," pulled from the website for the London-based Society of Analytical Psychology. For more information see www.thesap.org.

5 Jaffé 1971, p. 13.
6 von Franz 1975, p. 7.
7 The Society of Analytical Psychology, www.thesap.org, para. 2.
8 Moore 1992, p. xv.
9 Moore, 1992, p. xv.
10 Hillman 1972, p. 92.
11 Moore 1992, pp. 78–79.
12 Jung 1931a, para. 331.
13 For example, in the Platonic Dialogues Socrates admonishes Athenians for their shameful priorities. Instead of giving "attention or thought to truth and understanding and the perfection of soul," they devote their time to "acquiring as much money as possible" (Hamilton & Cairns 1961, p. 16). Placing the soul at the center of life, a religious endeavor, reappears in the work of the fifteenth century Neo-Platonist Marsilio Ficino, who "found soul to be the proper mediating factor in all his studies—in philosophy and theology, in medicine and psychotherapy, and in his religious devotion" (Moore 1982, p. 33). "There is indeed a relationship between soul and religion, between psychology and religious awareness," says Moore (1992), "for without soulful fantasy all is profane and secular, a world reduced to serve as fodder for our pragmatic intentions" (p. 44).
14 Jung 1960, para 343. The first paragraph of Jung's central essay on the nature of the psyche includes this remarkable sentence: "The history of psychology up to the seventeenth century consists essentially in the enumeration of doctrines concerning the soul, but the soul was never able to get a word in as the object investigated." Jung's statement is a textbook example of what James Hillman (1975) refers to as *personifying*, an attitude toward the psyche and psychic figures as autonomous and often eloquent persons. Personifying radically tilts psychology towards relationship *with* the psyche rather than analysis *of* it.
15 Moore 1994.
16 Ruszczynski & Fisher 1995, p. 118.
17 Rilke 1993, pp. 80–81.
18 Jung 1931a.
19 Freud 1912.
20 Jung 1946, para. 198.
21 Consider how Jung intentionally occupied two periods of history during his life as if he were a time traveler. In *Memories, Dreams, Reflections* (1961/1989), he describes slowly building his Tower at Bollingen as a solitary retreat a few miles from the Jung family home. Without leaving the shores of Lake Zurich, Jung could walk away from the twentieth century and inhabit the world of his medieval ancestors.
22 Jung 1946, para 529.
23 Some therapists, in addition to noticing patterns in human culture, develop an ecological sensibility. They become curious about transspecies behaviors and patterns, as well as the effects of the natural environment on patients, both of which express the idea that soul is in the world we inhabit.
24 Jung 1931b, para. 937.
25 From *The Divine Comedy* by Dante Alighieri 2000 [1321]. Translated by A. S. Kline. Copyright 2000–2002. Used with permission.
26 Cf. Edinger 1992, Jaffé 1971, Stein 1982, 1998, Storr 1983, Tacey 2012, von Franz 1975 & 1993, Yeoman & Lu 2024, and Young-Eisendrath & Dawson 1997.
27 Cf. Nell 2005.
28 Cf. Jung & Chodorow 1997.
29 Jung 1958.
30 Cf. Kalff 2003 [1966].

References

Alighieri, D. (2000). *The divine comedy* (A. S. Kline, Trans.). Poetry in Translation. https://www.poetryintranslation.com/klineasdante.php (Original work published ca. 1321.)

Corbett, L. (1996). *The religious function of the psyche.* Routledge.

Edinger, E. F. (1992). *Ego and archetype.* Shambhala.

Freud, S. (1912). Recommendations to physicians practising psycho-analysis. *SE* XII.

Hamilton, E., & Cairns, H. (Eds.) (1961). *The Collected Dialogues of Plato.* Princeton University Press.

Hillman, J. (1972). *The myth of analysis.* Northwestern University Press.

Hillman, J. (1975). *Re-visioning psychology.* HarperPerennial.

Jaffé, A. (1971). *The myth of meaning* (R. F. C. Hull, Trans.). G. P. Putnam's Sons.

Jung, C. G. (1931a). Marriage as a psychological relationship. *CW* 17.

Jung, C. G.(1931b). A psychological theory of types. *CW* 6.

Jung, C. G.(1946). The psychology of the transference. *CW* 16.

Jung, C. G.(1958). The transcendent function. *CW* 8.

Jung, C. G.(1960). On the nature of the psyche. *CW* 8.

Jung, C. G.(1989). *Memories, dreams, reflections* (A. Jaffé, Ed.; R. Winston & C. Winston, Trans.; Rev. edn). Vintage. (Original work published 1961.)

Jung, C. G., & Chodorow, J. (1997). *Jung on active imagination.* Princeton University Press.

Kalff, D. M. (2003). *Sandplay: A psychotherapeutic approach to the psyche.* Temenos Press. (Original work published 1966.)

Merriam-Webster. (n.d.). *Merriam Webster's collegiate dictionary.* Retrieved September 16, 2024. https://www.merriam-webster.com/dictionary/art.

Moore, T. (1982). *The planets within: The astrological psychology of Marsilio Ficino.* Lindisfarne Press.

Moore, T. (1992). *Care of the soul.* HarperPerennial.

Moore, T.(1994). *Soul mates.* HarperPerennial.

Nell, R. (2005). *The use of dreams in couple counseling* (D. Sharp, Ed.; S. Jellinghaus, Trans.). Inner City Books.

Nelson, E. É., & Delmedico, A. (2023). When left hands touch: shadow vows and Jung's quaternity. *Journal of Analytical Psychology*, 68(1), 48–70. https://doi.org/10.1111/1468-5922.12882.

Rilke, R. M. (1993). *Letters to a young poet* (S. Mitchell, Trans.). Shambhala.

Ruszczynski, S., & Fisher, J. (1995). *Intrusiveness and intimacy in the couple.* Routledge.

Society of Analytical Psychology. *What is the core of Jung's theory system?* https://www.thesap.org.uk/articles-on-jungian-psychology-2/carl-gustav-jung/.

Stein, M. (Ed.). (1982). *Jungian analysis.* Open Court.

Stein, M. (1998). *Jung's map of the soul.* Open Court.

Storr, A. (1983). *The essential Jung.* Princeton University Press.

Tacey, D. (2012). *The Jung reader.* Routledge.

von Franz, M.-L. (1975). *C. G. Jung speaking* (W. Kennedy, Trans.). Little, Brown & Company.

von Franz, M.-L. (1993). *Psychotherapy.* Shambhala.

Yeoman, A., & Lu, K. (2024). *C. G. Jung's collected works: The basics.* Routledge.

Young-Eisendrath, P., & Dawson, T. (Eds.). (1997). *The Cambridge companion to Jung.* Cambridge University Press.

Chapter 1

The Self, Individuation, and Jungian Couples Therapy

"First sentences are doorways to worlds," says Ursula Le Guin.[1] Although she was speaking of fiction, it is equally true of the first sentences of Jung's 1961 memoir, *Memories, Dreams, Reflections*. "My life is a story of the self-realization of the unconscious," he begins, "everything in the unconscious seeks outward manifestation, and the personality too desires to evolve out of its unconscious conditions and to experience itself as a whole."[2] In 37 words, Jung asserts the reality of the unconscious as an active, dynamic factor shaping the story of his life—not merely the passive counterpart to consciousness. Further, desire for wholeness drives psychological development. By the second paragraph of his memoir, Jung has rejected the language of science and its emphasis on general concepts and averages in favor of "the way of myth." People simply cannot experience themselves in numeric terms or diagnostic labels. We are so much more than that. Only myth grants us a vision of our lives that is particular and universal, time-bound and eternal.

For some psychotherapists, encountering the Jungian world is unsettling. For others, it is like returning home to recollect a forgotten language and reclaim a way of being that has been forced underground by Enlightenment rationality and its disfigured offspring, scientism. Many turn to Jungian thought because it is large enough to value the nonrational alongside the rational. They are inspired to trust intuitive insights alongside material evidence, to listen to the longings of the soul as a counterbalance to the agendas of the ego, and to cherish the deep, tender stories hidden within outward social roles and adaptive behaviors. Jung's ideas, like deep waters, have quietly risen through cracks in the bedrock certainties of mainstream psychology.

If first sentences are doorways to worlds, we might closely read how Jung introduces his world in fewer than three pages—even though his collected writing exceeds 18 thick volumes. Over the course of the memoir's evocative prologue, Jung expresses elements of a holistic worldview that has grown increasingly relevant since his death in 1961. His vision hearkens back to the ancient spiritual idea of an interconnected cosmos and it anticipates twenty-first century systems thinking in physics and the biological sciences. He sketches some large ideas, including humanity's relationship to the sacred and the

DOI: 10.4324/9781032688008-2

eternal, which may seem remote from the hands-on practice of couples therapy. Not so. The task of this chapter is to show how these ideas, and some of their nearest kin, form a meaningful approach to partners suffering in relationship.

The Archetype of Wholeness, the Self

"Like every other being, I am a splinter of the infinite deity" Jung says in the prologue to his memoir, "a psychic process [I] do not control, or only partly direct."[3] Jung is alluding to the Self, the archetype of wholeness that orchestrates the process of growth towards wholeness. "It might equally well be called the 'God within us,'" he says, since "the beginnings of our whole psychic life seem to be inextricably rooted in this point, and all our highest and ultimate purposes seem to be striving towards it."[4] Embedded in these images is a paradox. The Self is a splinter and a point, "the smallest of the small, easily overlooked and pushed aside."[5] And it is the whole of the person's life, the largest, the highest, the ultimate, the totality. Jungian thought is replete with such paradoxes, and Jung does not attempt to resolve them. The important element for psychotherapy is just this: the couple's conscious motivation for seeking help is only *part* of the story. What may be emerging is an unconscious longing or need directed by the Self. The Self, the god within, urges partners toward wholeness—and therapists are a part of that process.

The process of self-realization is realization of the Self. As Jungian analyst Erich Neumann points out, the awareness of the reality of one's entire Self ousts the ego "from its central position in a psyche organised on the lines of a monarchy or totalitarian state;" its place is "taken by wholeness or the self, which is now recognised as central."[6] What does the centrality of the Self mean in practice? For many people it may begin with a painful loss of control, a confrontation with intense emotions that suddenly erupt, or fateful events that appear to happen out of nowhere. The ego becomes powerless and comfortable social roles turn out to be the cloak and the shell covering a far more complex personality. Some parts are likeable, and some parts are not: intimate relationship reveals both.

Jung introduced the term *shadow* to describe aspects of the whole personality people dismiss, ignore, or repress. Working with the shadow is the first step on the journey toward wholeness, the first encounter with the power of the Self which, Jung says, always defeats the ego:

> The self, in its efforts at self-realization, reaches out beyond the ego-personality on all sides; because of its all-encompassing nature it is brighter and darker than the ego, and accordingly confronts it with problems which it would like to avoid. Either one's moral courage fails, or one's insight, or both, until in the end fate decides. ... For this reason, the experience of the self is always a defeat for the ego.[7]

That defeat for the ego-personality—often manifesting in partners as the failure to make the relationship work, or to get what they want or need from their partner, or the evaporation of tenderness, respect, joy, and sexual excitement—is nearly inconceivable for people with a strong will. They are more accustomed to solving problems, asserting control, or achieving success through sheer effort. The Self erupts with the first, startling intimation that something else, something not-yet-known, is going on, and it is well beyond the ego's control. Jungian couples therapists recognize such goings-on as the presence of the unconscious psyche.

Over time, partners begin to recognize the subtle impulses from the unconscious as nudges towards wholeness. The Self as center point becomes the goal of psychic development, a kind of orienting device that might show up as an inner figure or a dream motif that continues to be persistent and purposeful. "There is no linear evolution; there is only circumambulation of the self," Jung realized while observing himself and his patients; "uniform development exists, at most, only at the beginning; later, everything points toward the center."[8]

Becoming oneself is not a solitary process. The realization of the Self requires relationship, both public, social relationship with objectively real people and relationship with inner guides or figures. "You can never come to your self by building a meditation hut on top of Mount Everest; you will only be visited by your own ghosts and that is not individuation," Jung says, because "the self appears in your deeds and deeds always mean relationship."[9] How better to see your whole self—expressed in thought, word, and deed, for better and for worse—than in an emotionally committed relationship? Certainly, partners adopt roles with one another, but home life is also where social masks drop voluntarily or crack under pressure, involuntarily.

In summary, for Jung, the aim of individual life is wholeness. Couples therapists might begin by wondering how their work with troubled partners serves the Self. Is it the Self who has brought the couple to the threshold of your office and, in all likelihood, to a threshold moment in the relationship? What wants to be known? Jung offers another image in the Prologue to *Memories, Dreams, Reflections* which may evoke an answer to these poignant and difficult questions:

> Life has always seemed to me like a plant that lives on its rhizome. Its true life is invisible, hidden in the rhizome. The part that appears above ground lasts only a single summer. ... Yet I have never lost a sense of something that endures underneath the eternal flux.[10]

Following this image, couples therapists can think of themselves as gardeners during the winter of their patients' discontent, trusting that the barren surface is not the whole story. Working below, in the depths, therapists help couples discover the healthy rhizome in need of tending.

Working with Images

Readers of Jung notice how often he turns to images to express important ideas. He thought of images as the soul's own language. "Everything of which we are conscious is an image ... image is psyche."[11] Jung realized that images are not flat or two-dimensional pictures, like the photos people see in a magazine, collect on their smartphones, or post on social media. Jung found that psychic images are three-dimensional and full of soul, which refers to their interiority and expressive power. They can be captivating or memorable images from waking life (animals, persons, trees, canyons, or rivers); last night's dream of an animal, a person, a tree, a canyon, a river; objects (a coffee cup, a blanket); or a multi-sensory environment (a redwood forest, a room, an office building).

A good example of image-as-environment is the setting where therapy takes place. Many therapists already realize their clinical office is a revealing environment, artfully arranged to provide an embodied felt sense of the work that accumulates slowly from session to session. To deepen their sense of the setting, therapists can ask, *How does my therapy office evoke soul?* Try to see and feel the environment freshly. Note the lighting and temperature. Note the colors and textures of walls and furnishings and the selection and arrangement of meaningful pictures, paintings, and objects on display. All of it taken together as a gestalt is a rich and generative image. It, too, tells a story.

The interiority and soulfulness of images may seem odd to some readers, but you might play with the idea first in your own life and then with couples. Partners naturally use metaphors when describing their issues—and, at the core of every metaphor is an image. For example, suppose a partner describes feeling suffocated in the relationship. Instead of just adding it to the list of complaints, therapists can pause and express curiosity, particularly if there is something about suffocation that captures their imagination. They can ask, *This feeling of suffocation, how do you mean it? What is it like for you?* Here, it is important for the therapist to pause and wait patiently for a response because this type of question kindles the wounded psyche to produce an image—a metaphor for what is going on and how serious it is. If an image is not forthcoming, the therapist can prompt the psyche by asking further questions: *Is it like a hand on your throat? A bag over your head? How do you mean it?* Again, the therapist waits. The partner's psyche will then realize it is being invited into the conversation and the partner will usually respond with some personal authority and newly discovered inner knowing. They might say, for example, *No, it's not like any of those. It's more like I'm stuck in a tiny little box with no air holes and can't get out.* Now the therapist has an image to explore, and can turn to the other partner who, while listening, has had to contend with their own reactions, and ask them: *And what about you? Did you know that your partner was suffocating and stuck in a tiny box? I wonder, are you suffocating, too? In a box?* The partner's psyche will usually respond with a different image, helping the couple notice more clearly how they are experiencing their relationship.

A couple's images shift and change as new metaphors come forth. All are bellwethers for how their therapy is proceeding. Fundamentally, working with images as expressive emissaries with something to offer—intuitive insights or feelings, another way of seeing or imagining—enlivens therapy. It is like conversation with a friend who is helping guide the work.

Wait, what? Talk with an image? Yes, though you might simply begin by observing the image for a while, noticing how it changes, grows, moves, or expresses itself. Jung's own dreams indicated that images are alive. For instance, he dreamed of a twelfth-century crusader in chainmail lying upon a sarcophagus, hands clasped. Then, in what must have been a spooky moment, Jung saw a finger of the stony left hand "beginning to stir."[12] He reports this and other dreams during a momentous turning point in his life, when he began to discover his own psychological ground by letting himself descend into the images. Jung remained devoted to this process all his life. As James Hillman points out, Jung's devotion to his images rather than orthodox religion or prevailing psychological theory boldly demonstrates Jung's faith in the psyche.[13]

Jungian couples therapy welcomes images as alive and full of meaning. For instance, one partner may describe a meaningful dream image from long ago, perhaps related to their first date. Or perhaps a pivotal moment in the relationship takes on the qualities of a tableau, something like a waking dream image that dramatizes an emotional truth. Without apparent cause, and in a short span of time, reminders of the image might then appear everywhere: in casual conversation, on billboards, in social media, on the cover of a magazine. The weirdly omnipresent image is captivating *as if* it wants attention. In a psychological sense it is alive.

The Residue of the Past and the Pull of the Future

A great deal of excellent therapy traces a couple's suffering to families of origin. Such an historical view was Freud's abiding interest, as his psychology grounded in the Oedipal myth suggests.[14] The elaboration of psychoanalysis by Melanie Klein and others who formed the object relations school likewise placed strong emphasis on the residue of childhood experience in the immediate family, describing how the child internalized objects, which then populated their internal world long into adulthood.[15] The emphasis on formative childhood experience is also apparent in mid-century attachment theory, which focuses on potent, durable emotional patterns arising first between child and caregiver, as described in the work of Mary Ainsworth and John Bowlby.[16] Contemporary findings in neuroscience on the persistence of early childhood neural patterning, for instance in the work of Daniel Siegel, Alan Schore, and Bessel van der Kolk, strongly supports attachment theory.[17] Sue Johnson's emotionally focused therapy (EFT), a fruitful counterpart to cognitive-behaviorism, prioritizes understanding childhood attachment patterns.[18]

Therapists often explore the social roles and attachment patterns that shape how partners live together and love each other. There is little question that partners' portraits of ideal love relationships are flavored by how they were, or were not, loved as children. Partners hope to recapitulate (or create for the first time) the oceanic feelings of blissful, friction-free union idealized between mother (or maternal figure) and child. Exploring the impact of the intrusion of reality on these fantasies is integral to couples therapy, something expanded upon in the exploration in Chapter 5 of the shadows of the vows that couples make when joining together.

A Jungian approach to couples therapy, however, does not literalize childhood by focusing exclusively on memories and relational patterns in the family of origin from twenty, thirty, or forty years ago. The past, in Jungian thought, also includes the millennia-old ancestral heritage of our species, the collective unconscious or objective psyche. These "historical layers" are not "just dead dust, but alive and continuously active in everyone."[19] The past also includes cultural and family history, comprising childhood patterns, beliefs, and trauma that can also have a transgenerational origin, which are equally alive and continuously active.

Beyond Jung's expansive notion of the past, his theory of individuation departs significantly, yet subtly, from the therapeutic focus on family-of-origin issues. It recognizes that every person's life stretches between two poles, past and future. Of course, the past is remembered and endlessly repeated through established patterns of thought, belief, and behavior. Yet just as influential, according to Jung, is the pull of the future, which is guided by the Self, the archetype of wholeness described above. Jung, noting the alienation and fragmentation of contemporary life, the loss of meaning and mystery, asserted the crucial importance of the Self. It is both the orienting center of psychological life and its circumference, something like a home for the soul, which "can live only in and from human relationships."[20] By asserting the purposefulness of life however it is expressed, couples are invited to look not only to old patterns and wounding, but also to what is emerging. Deep examination frequently results in the painful yet quite necessary individuation of one or both partners. The presence of the Self in the work can sustain couples through periods of despair and confusion as well as sustain couples therapists through periods of professional self-doubt.

Jung asserts that "individuation is an ineluctable psychological necessity."[21] It is also a never-ending process that frequently means the call to particular kinds of relationships. Some devoted couples reject the legal institution of marriage while it is important to others. Some prefer same-sex partners while others are drawn to people of the opposite sex, and some enjoy both. Contemporary coupling, the subject of Chapter 7, reveals many varied forms and styles of intimacy—as well as the need for solitude within relationship. The work of individuation follows no preconceived pattern, form, or timetable, nor can therapy force one upon it.

There are also other types of relationships necessary for individuation. These can include one's commitments outside of the partnership, a theme touched upon in Chapter 5. They may draw the person's *eros*, or life energy, away from coupled life. These relationships include passionate commitment to a profession, a cause, one's own creative work, a style of life, or an activity, and they can be as demanding as human partnership.

The Collective Unconscious

In the earliest decades of Jung's professional career, human knowledge was divided into well-defended disciplines. These intellectual silos persisted to the point where expertise required an increasingly narrow focus that persists to this day.[22] As Tacey points out, however, "knowledge which continues to fragment the world, to separate humanity from nature, to split spirit from earth and mind from body, is being viewed with a new kind of suspicion."[23] In this, as in so many other things, Jung was far ahead of his time. He was a radically transgressive thinker and, in an era striving to make psychology into a reductive science, he was "the idealistic and romantic explorer of the mind, always looking for traces of the sacred" in everyday life.[24]

From natural inclination and the need to establish a firm foundation for his approach to psyche and Self, Jung sought an objective source for his analytical psychology. Psychological theory drawn from his personal clinical experience was simply not enough. As he listened to the dreams of his patients, Jung saw "the analogies between dream-images and universal mythological motifs,"[25] which prompted one of Jung's distinctive contributions to psychology: the idea of the collective unconscious, or the objective psyche. Jung asserts that modern people are rooted in an ancestral lineage of ideas, behaviors, beliefs, stories, and images. Just as the body carries vestiges of its ancient past in bone and blood, representing "a whole museum of organs with its long evolutionary history behind them," so too, the mind is "organized in a similar way."[26] The mind, via imagination and recollection, carries our instinctual, cultural, and spiritual past. However the mind is defined—a question of intense debate and interest among neuroscientists and others—it is not local. Neither is it personal.[27] Rather, mind includes species memory reflecting the human history of instinctual needs, spiritual aspirations, and creative outpourings.

The Way of Myth

From our earliest utterances and cave etchings, there has always been an instinct for humans to tell the story of their relationship to the world and to each other. We express our beliefs and values, what we love, what we hate, what we fear—because more than *homo sapiens* we are *homo faber* or man the maker—and we exist within the stories we make. "Perhaps stories are so much a part of us because human life itself has the structure of story," says veteran journalist Jack Lule; "each of us has a central character. Each of us knows, better than we know anything, that life has a beginning, middle, and end. We need stories because we are stories."[28]

Thinking of ourselves as storytelling animals brings us to another key point in the prologue to Jung's memoir. In the end, all of us must find the particular myth that helps us make sense of our lives. That myth is often *numinous*, a word Jung borrowed from theologian and philosopher Rudolf Otto, meaning something that has an unforgettable emotional impact.[29] These stories, figures, memories, symbols, and images have an inexhaustible life that never reveal themselves fully but continue to nourish us in new ways. We return to them again and again—or they show up with uncanny timing—at which point we often respond with a sense of familiarity (*Ah, you again!*), surprise (*What's up now?* or *What's the story?*), or kindness (*Welcome back, friend*).

Jung's psychology draws from classical philosophy, including the rationalism of Plato and Aristotle as well as humanity's spiritual longing expressed in Greek epic literature, poetry, and drama. "Myth lives vividly in our symptoms and fantasies and in our conceptual systems" and gives our concepts "their vitality and credibility. Mythology is a psychology of antiquity. Psychology is a mythology of modernity."[30] The vitality and numinosity of a couple's story—indeed, their personal myth—shows up when they tell it with tremendous energy and conviction. Working with couples to root their story in a more encompassing mythic sensibility is like hearing it as a motif played to an ancient tune. It helps foster a healthy psychological curiosity and imaginative engagement so couples enter more deeply into the mystery and meaning of their relationship. Awareness of "the eternal drama" of myth adds a dimension to existence "usually reserved for the poets."[31] It transposes the questions of life from a personal to a transpersonal mode and inspires culturally imaginative reflection. Though couples' stories are quite personal, mythic reflection can depersonalize conflict(s) just enough to re-seat them in larger contexts. Even a small shift in perspective can relieve suffering and create deeper understanding.

Developing a mythic sensibility also enriches professional practice and personal life. It is essential to the soulful dimensions of therapy, and it returns therapy to its original meaning, care of the soul, discussed later in the chapter. It is not possible to place the soul at the center of the therapeutic endeavor—the souls of the partners, the soul of the relationship, and the therapist's own soul—without an appreciation of myth. Mythological images, including archetypal figures, motifs, and scenarios, give therapists ways of understanding the rich complexity of human life. The conscious mind, without appreciation of myth, "will have no bridge to the deeper psychic layers."[32] Mythology roots us in the eternal drama, helping therapists and couples regard the clinical hour creatively as *poesis*, a making.

Excursion: Jung and the DSM

The first edition of the *Diagnostic and Statistical Manual of Mental Disorders* (DSM) was published in 1952. Since its initial appearance, it has grown from a scant 32 pages describing 106 conditions to nearly 1,000 pages precisely categorizing nearly 300 mental disorders identified through acceptable scientific procedures. Undoubtedly an excellent compendium of useful information, the DSM may also have an unfortunate consequence antithetical to soul. There is a conceit in minds inhospitable to mystery, overly dominated by reason, and convinced of one's manipulative powers: the erroneous belief that by merely naming a thing, one has understood the thing.

Jung was known in his field and could have been on the DSM's editorial board, collaborating with other psychiatrists concerned with psychopathology. Instead, his mind was engaged in the deepest layers of human experience, exploring subjects as varied as contemporary religion and quantum physics. Thus, at a time when the American Psychiatric Association was categorizing mental disorders, Jung's intellect was on display in his 1951 work, *Aion*, which describes the phenomenology of the Self, dismantling conventional views of space–time in "Synchronicity, an acausal connecting principle," and debating good, evil, and the character of Yahweh in *Answer to Job*.

To say that Jung's interests did not lie in composing a technical manual is quite the understatement. Even if Jung had been invited to contribute to the DSM, he doubtless would have declined the offer. He makes his predilection clear in *Aion* when he says "in describing the living processes of the psyche, I deliberately and consciously give preference to a dramatic, mythological way of thinking and speaking. Because this is not only more expressive but also more exact than an abstract scientific terminology."[33]

Jung's abiding interest in a mythological way of thinking and speaking directly applies to coupled life. Relationships are mysteries to be lived. They cannot be reduced, generalized, and abstracted. Jung alludes to the limitations of diagnostic language by asserting that "the intellectual 'grasp' of a psychological fact produces no more than a concept of it" which is "no more than a name, a *flatus vocis*."[34] He describes such labels as "intellectual counters" easily bandied about, passing "lightly from hand to hand, for they have no weight or substance. They sound full but are hollow; and though purporting to designate a heavy task and obligation, they commit us to nothing."[35] The language of soul is much weightier. It comes slowly, sometimes after a long, gestating silence, if it comes at all. Such halting attempts reflect the therapist's or couple's struggle to describe carefully the embodied felt sense of what is going on. As therapists attuned to somatics realize, speaking the truth lodged deeply in one's own flesh is often the genuine beginning of transformation.

Helping couples find and speak the language of the soul is immensely difficult for everyone at first. Therapists can gently foster the process by keeping an eye and ear tuned to the metaphors in the couples' language, as well as paying attention to the images that arise in them while

listening. Jung reiterates the value of imagery in *Answer to Job*, possibly his most controversial work since it deals directly with religious belief. The only way he could speak of Job's deep mysteries was to "move in a world of images that point to something ineffable."[36] In Jung's late great work on alchemy, *Mysterium Coniunctionis*, published a few years after *Answer to Job*, he again affirms the value of images. "Concepts are coined and negotiable values; images are life."[37]

Jung on Relationship

A consistent theme in contemporary Jungian couples theory is the description of relationships as a challenging path for individuation.[38] This theory draws from Jung's 1925 essay "Marriage as a Psychological Relationship." Conventional couples rarely challenge the inherited traditions of their families of origin, although they may chafe from time to time against unspoken cultural and religious rules. Mostly, conventional relationships may be lived quietly, in relative comfort. In psychological relationships, couples are more conscious of themselves as individuals and of how they participate in and create the partnership from day to day. They notice—or, more often, stumble painfully over—the familial and cultural forces that have shaped their roles, expectations, and fantasies of coupled life. Psychological relationships are a perilous endeavor. When conventional patterns of relating break down, and couples can no longer ignore their conflicts or withstand the old, usual ways of being together, their souls may be demanding a new psychological relationship.

Jung notes that emotionally committed relationships and individuation are interrelated and entwined. (It is as though marriage, too, was part of Jung's lifelong psychological education.) First, consciousness as an individual requires distinguishing oneself from others and standing apart from the beliefs, assumptions, and biases of family and culture; in short, agonizing separation from one's inherited traditions. Commitment to a partner is likely to be someone's first adult choice to immerse themselves in a psychologically alien environment. It should be no surprise that partners show up for therapy bewildered and disoriented. As Haule puts it, falling in love "draws us away from our family of origin" and "brings us face to face with a soul more foreign than any we have known, and yet marked with an uncanny familiarity."[39] It is often accompanied by the "conviction that we were 'meant' to meet or that we have known one another in a former life" which reveals the "archetypal power of the encounter."[40] Second, people who remain partly or wholly enmeshed in their family of origin are likely to choose a mate in a "purely instinctive" fashion, which produces "only a kind of impersonal liaison."[41]

A psychological relationship can only take place when there is a clearer distinction between oneself and another. Partners discover and develop more of their unique identities, which often begins with exploring the shadow. "The young person of marriageable age," (or anyone who is unconscious or psychologically naïve) "is certain to have wide areas which still live in the shadow."[42] Regardless of the level of consciousness, people making a commitment to a beloved always start with at least some degree of naïveté. Partners willing to confront their shadow and examine deeper elements of their psyches follow the challenging path of individuation to create a psychological relationship together.

After Jung describes the challenges of a psychological relationship, he develops his theory of the container and the contained. Here, he falls into the gender essentialism that feminists have also discovered elsewhere in his writings. As an example, Jung wrote, "it is an almost a regular occurrence for a woman to be wholly contained, spiritually, in her husband, and for a husband to be wholly contained, emotionally, in his wife."[43] This observation neatly splits couples into separate domains of expertise that recapitulate old, tired debates about innate gender-specific skills, e.g., *men don't do emotion* and *women aren't capable of abstract thought.* A partner who is contained, Jung adds, lives almost entirely within the confines of the relationship with "no essential obligations and no binding interests" outside of it.[44] He regards this as an ideal partnership save for one "unpleasant side ... the disquieting dependence upon a personality that can never be seen in its entirety."[45]

Jung's theory reveals a problematic supposition beyond the gender essentialism that went unquestioned in mid-twentieth-century thinking. Regardless of who is the container and who is the contained, the personality of *either* partner can never be seen in its entirety. Individuation is a ceaseless psychological process with many twists and turns. Each partner is a mystery to each other *and* to themselves, which means the relationship, too, is fundamentally mysterious. It can only be lived, which is a most unnerving idea for couples seeking predictability. The idea that their souls are deeply interfused in the relationship, and that relationship may be necessary to their individuation, is altogether more unnerving. This approach is postmodern, non-hierarchical, co-created, and grounded in mutuality. As any experienced therapist knows, creating a more conscious relationship is immense and painful psychological work.

Jung's essay on marriage and individuation appears in Volume 17 of the *Collected Works*. The title of the volume, *The Development of Personality*, can be misleading for contemporary readers since personality does not adequately express what Jung meant at the time. The twenty-first century has seen a full flowering of the cult of personality and the rise of social media influencers, both of which carry a whiff of egoistic superficiality. A word closer to Jung's meaning is *character*—which has more weight, substance, integrity, and depth. Personality can be performed; character is revealed. This distinction may account for a paradox in couples therapy: as therapist and couple turn their attention to the soul of the relationship, each partner grows more substantial as an individual, more fully integrated as themselves. In some cases, of course, it may lead to the end of a relationship, particularly if one or both partners arrived on the therapist's doorstep mentally, emotionally, and materially ready for the end. But in a surprising number of cases, the growth in character of each partner individually can create a sturdier, more substantial, and more satisfying union. In the words of Rainer Maria Rilke, if "a wonderful living side-by-side" emerges, a couple may succeed in "loving the distance between them which makes it possible for each to see the other whole and against a wide sky."[46]

The Necessity of Relationship?

For some couples, their souls may demand profound and intimate relationship in order to grow toward wholeness. Partners may enter therapy feeling the weight of this demand, but with little idea how to remain committed—or even whether preserving their relationship is the right choice. Or they may have little idea that intimate relationship is one of the ways their souls find expression, as tumultuous and painful as it frequently is. Yet some Jungian analysts assert the *psychological* necessity of a profound, committed relationship with another human being.

For example, Marie-Louise von Franz, Jung's long-time colleague and the translator of alchemical texts, called the wedding ring "a connection and a fetter."[47] Even so, the dreams of her patients indicated that "the marriage has to be made for the sake of individuation."[48] It is as if their souls realize the full weight of the commitment, even if the ego is unaware or, in painful moments of conflict, seeks a way out. Adolph Guggenbühl-Craig, another prominent Jungian analyst, viewed marriage as an *opus contra naturam* that creates trouble, not happiness. It is a "special path for discovering soul," both "evasionless" and "tormenting."[49] The legal accessibility of divorce today opens avenues of escape for those who choose to separate. If the troubles in the current relationship are not addressed, they often resurface in some form or fashion in future ones. While individuals can attempt to ignore the deeper psychological conflicts that erupt with one partner, they will never be free of them until, for the sake of individuation, they work through them.[50]

For embattled partners just beginning couples therapy, striving for wholeness may be the furthest things from their mind, union only a distant memory with no chance of return. By remaining attentive to the sacred, whole-making dimension of their relationship, the couple may come to view their suffering differently and "stake one's whole being" on the difficult work of individuation. "Nothing less will do; there can be no easier conditions, no substitutes, no compromises."[51]

Intimate partnership is an especially potent opportunity for individuation because it is often the first relationship partners voluntarily choose. "We let down our boundaries and allow ourselves to penetrate and be penetrated by another person ... learn new ways to say, 'help me,' and we listen for our partner's cry."[52] A couple's suffering may ultimately prove to be transformative. The medieval poet John Gower described it exquisitely: "*Est amor egra salus, vexata quies, pius error, bellica pax, vulnus dulce, suave malum*" (Love is a sharp salvation, a troubled quiet, a pious error, a warring peace, a sweet wound, a soothing ill).[53] It takes great moral courage to expose one's wounds to the gaze of another. Yet it is a sweet achievement.

Couples Therapy as Care of the Soul

Jung listened carefully to the spiritual longings of his patients and welcomed their expression as essential to the healing process. In fact, central to Jung's thinking about the psyche is a reverence for esoteric traditions that recognized the correspondence between inner and outer, matter and spirit, personal and transpersonal—the fundamental relatedness of all things and beings. Yet he withstood withering criticism from other psychotherapists and psychoanalysts, many of whom dismissed spirituality and were deaf to soul. Readers of Jung's work, however, appreciate this emphasis on the search for meaning and the cultivation of soul, both of which help to relieve suffering.

Therapists can tend spiritual elements that emerge in the work by noticing what is numinous for each partner or the couple. During a numinous experience, one "is in contact with something that is 'wholly other,' beyond the sphere of what is usual, intelligible and familiar."[54] The numinous is often found in long-held secrets, things patients reveal to therapists only with great trepidation. Attending to what is numinous allows therapists to work with deeply spiritual matters found at the heart of suffering. The clinical space is enriched by conversation about meaning and its loss, just as it is enriched by listening to the soul's longing for something mysterious and unnamable. Attuning to the soul of a relationship can be likened to tracing a meandering path through a dark forest, always listening at the edge where the known and the unknown meet.

Prioritizing spiritual experience and care of the soul in couples therapy alters many things, perhaps especially the meaning of suffering. Suffering is evidence that the Self, the archetype of wholeness who guides the individuation process, is active in the relationship. A soul psychology emphasizes a third space between the spiritual and the physical.[55] Historically, couples therapy has focused upon making physical (behavioral) moves to help couples reunite or trying to help couples transcend their problems in the effort to reunite spiritually. Since most couples come to therapy in need of both physical and spiritual renewal, it is easy to neglect the third place, the *soul* of the relationship where symptoms lie festering. Because of pain or fear, it is also the place couples try to avoid. Therapists will notice this aversion when couples come to therapy in the aftermath of an affair. One partner may be wholly committed to *putting the past behind us, so we can move forward*, while the other partner needs a full reckoning. Betrayal creates a spiritual crisis in which one or both partners question their beliefs about all they held to be true and sacred. The numinous core of the wound invites them back, time and again, for a more complete working through.

To actively embrace suffering as a necessity imposed by the Self requires faith in the slow, mysterious processes of transformation. Such faith is radically countercultural because it challenges the Western fantasy of cure and control. Care of the soul, by contrast, "isn't about curing, fixing, changing, adjusting" or restoring the partners or the relationship to so-called health so that they can enjoy a trouble-free future, says Thomas Moore, guided by "some idea of perfection or even improvement." [56] Rather, therapy as a spiritual practice, on behalf of soul, "remains patiently in the present, close to life as it presents itself day by day." [57] Although such a guiding aim may seem too modest, as though the therapist is doing little during the hour, nothing could be further from the truth. Finding the right words, "words that carry soul accurately, where thought, image, and feeling interweave" is "a miracle ... the most complex psychic endeavor imaginable." [58]

The Transferential Field of Couples Therapy

In Jung's essay on the problems of modern psychotherapy, he admits, "there are no universally valid recipes and rules ... only individual cases" that involve "the whole being of the doctor." [59] However, one universal phenomenon serves as the foundation of therapeutic work: the transference. Transference refers to the relationship between therapist and patients in which each influences the other through the projection of unconscious contents. Unconscious contents are transferred onto the therapist and, in turn, the therapist projects their unconscious contents onto patients (countertransference). In a very short time, transference and countertransference create an intense psychological bond. Human connection, Jung says, "is the core of the whole transference phenomenon, and it is impossible to argue it away." [60] Dissatisfaction between partners may stem from their transference projections onto one another. Therapists help couples become more conscious of these transferences in order to clear up misperceptions about one another and the distortions in their communications.

Psychoanalytic descriptions of the relational field within which couples therapy takes place also use the terms transference, countertransference, and projection. Fundamentally, they serve to draw the therapist into the unfolding drama. The couple's distress, like psyche's images, compels participation and stirs the therapist's own memories, wounds, and fantasies about relationships and commitment. Many therapists report uncanny similarities between their patients' emotional history and their own, which can indicate the strength of the therapist's countertransference and an invitation for them to rework old wounding. The therapeutic container, in other words, can get very hot very quickly—a frequent and difficult aspect of couples work that is not conveyed by cool technical vocabulary and training vignettes. (In fact, one wonders whether cool technical language is a defense against the heat of therapy.) In the transferential field shared by therapist and couple—albeit experienced differently by each—fantasies and memories dance together, a lively and living process.

The transferential field, the shared atmosphere of the work, is ever-changing. Jung points out that its volatility has a purpose: revelation. Working with the volatile content of the field *is* the therapy. It is also a shared somatic field in which much more than talk is going on. Each person is a whole, unique, expressive body. Each *says* much more than they *speak* via posture, gesture, breathing, facial expressions, as well as moving closer to one another or retreating. Couples are often aware of what is going on between them somatically but rarely have the ability to slow down and talk about it. Attuned therapists notice these somatic shifts, some quite subtle, and help partners voice the messages implicit in them.

Therapists are familiar with the volatility of couples work and know just how tricky it can be to maintain one's embodied, empathetic presence in the face of it. Capturing the quintessence of the therapist–patient relationship, Jung writes, "when two chemical substances combine, both are altered."[61] This statement applies equally well to suffering couples: they have combined their lives, they have altered each other. Even if partners decide to separate, their souls, like two volatile substances, continue to interact.

Despite the emphasis on individual therapy in Jungian analytic practice, Jungian thought is well-suited for couples work. Jung's emphasis on lifelong psychological transformation rooted in ongoing relationship with the unconscious offers an artful way of imagining the fluid, creative, and ultimately mysterious process of individuation. By highlighting the Self, Jung offers couples and therapists a nuanced framework to reimagine love's difficulties as valuable psychospiritual moments, full of soul. Jungian couple therapy cultivates the emerging wholeness of each partner, their relationship, and, indeed, the courageous therapist who guides them.

Notes

1 Le Guin 1989, p. 213.
2 Jung 1989[1961], p. 3.
3 Jung 1989[1961], p. 4.
4 Jung 1966, para. 399.
5 Jung 1959, para. 257.
6 Neumann 1990[1969], p. 18.
7 Jung 1963, para. 778.
8 Jung 1989[1961], pp. 196–197.
9 Jung 1988, pp. 794–795.

10 Jung 1989[1961], p. 4.
11 Jung 1967, para. 75.
12 Jung 1989[1961], p. 173.
13 Hillman 1983.
14 Freud 1989[1960].
15 Klien 1984[1975].
16 Cf. Ainsworth & Wall 2015 and Bowlby 1988.
17 Cf. Siegal 2012, Schore 2012, and van der Kolk 2015.
18 Johnson 2019.
19 Jung 1950, para. 712.
20 Jung 1946, para. 444.
21 Jung 1966, para. 241.
22 Some scholars are actively attempting to transcend the sturdy walls of knowledge silos by practicing *intersectionality*. Psychologists talk to sociologists, anthropologists, historians, philosophers, physicists, philologists, biologists, neuroscientists, and many, many others—with the aim of a more holistic understanding of the human experience. Faced with the immense and complex problems of the twenty-first century, we must talk to each other now more than ever.
23 Tacey 2012, p. 18.
24 Tacey 2012, p. 8.
25 Jung 1976, para. 522.
26 Jung 1967, para. 522.
27 Cf. Damasio 1999, 2010 and Zimmer 2004.
28 Lule 2001, p. 4.
29 Otto 1936.
30 Hillman 1979, pp. 23–24.
31 Edinger 1994, p. 3.
32 Edinger 1994, p. 2.
33 Jung 1951, para. 25.
34 Jung 1959, para. 60.
35 Jung 1959, para. 60.
36 Jung 1952, para. 555.
37 Jung 1963, para. 226.
38 Nelson & Delmedico 2023.
39 Haule 1984, p. iv.
40 Haule 1984, p. iv.
41 Jung 1925, para. 329.
42 Jung 1925, para. 327.
43 Jung 1925, para. 331c.
44 Jung 1925, para. 332.
45 Jung 1925, para. 332.
46 Rilke 1975, p. 28.
47 von Franz 1970, p. 58.
48 von Franz 1970, p. 58.
49 Guggenbühl-Craig 1977, pp. 41–42.
50 Freud 1914.
51 Jung 1939, para. 906.
52 Solfvin 1989, p. 101.
53 Gower 1857[1390], p. 42.
54 Corbett 1996, p. 12.
55 Hillman 1975, pp. 67–68.
56 Moore 1992, p. xv.

57 Moore 1992, p. xv.
58 Hillman 1975, p. 217.
59 Jung 1931, para. 163.
60 Jung 1946, para. 445. Jung asserts that the transferential relationship fosters the individuation of the couple *and* the therapist, adding in the same paragraph, "Relationship to the [S]elf is at once relationship to our fellow man, and no one can be related to the latter until he is related to himself."
61 Jung 1946, para 358.

References

Ainsworth, M., & Wall, S. (2015). *Patterns of attachment*. Routledge.

Bowlby, J. (1988). *Attachment and loss*. Basic Books.

Corbett, L. (1996). *The religious function of the psyche*. Routledge.

Damasio, A. (1999). *The feeling of what happens*. Harcourt Brace.

Damasio, A.(2010). *Self comes to mind*. Pantheon.

Edinger, E. (1994). *The eternal drama*. Shambhala.

Freud, S. (1914). Remembering, repeating, and working-through. *SE* XII.

Freud, S.(1989). *Introductory lectures on psychoanalysis*. Liveright. (Original work published 1960.)

Gower, J. (1857). *Confessio amantis*, Vol. I (R. Pauli, Ed.). Bell and Daldy. (Original work published 1390.)

Guggenbühl-Craig, A. (1977). *Marriage: Dead or alive* (M. Stein, Trans.). Spring Publications.

Haule, J. (1984). Foreword. In R. Stein, *The betrayal of the soul in psychotherapy* (2nd edn) (pp. *i–xiii*). Spring Journal Books.

Hillman, J. (1975). *Re-Visioning psychology*. HarperPerennial.

Hillman, J.(1979). *The dream and the underworld*. Harper & Row.

Hillman, J.(1983). *Healing fiction*. Spring Publications.

Johnson, S. (2019). *Emotionally-focused couple therapy* (3rd edn). Routledge.

Jung, C. G. (1925). Marriage as a psychological relationship. *CW* 17.

Jung, C. G.(1931). Problems of modern psychotherapy. *CW* 16.

Jung, C. G.(1939). Foreword to Suzuki's "Introduction to Zen Buddhism."*CW* 11.

Jung, C. G.(1946). The psychology of the transference. *CW* 16.

Jung, C. G.(1950). Concerning mandala symbolism. *CW* 9i.

Jung, C. G.(1959). Aion: Researches into the phenomenology of the Self. *CW* 9ii.

Jung, C. G.(1952). *Answer to Job*. *CW* 11.

Jung, C. G.(1963). *Mysterium Coniunctionis*. *CW* 14.

Jung, C. G.(1966). Two essays on Analytical Psychology. *CW* 7.

Jung, C. G.(1967). Commentary on "The secret of the golden flower."*CW* 13.

Jung, C. G.(1976). The symbolic life. *CW* 18.

Jung, C. G.(1988). *Nietzsche's Zarathustra* (J. Jarrett, Ed.). Princeton University Press.

Jung, C. G.(1989). *Memories, dreams, reflections* (A. Jaffé, Ed.; R. Winston & C. Winston, Trans.; Rev. edn). Vintage. (Original work published 1961.)

Klein, M. (1984). *The psychoanalysis of children* (J. Strachey, Trans.). The Free Press. (Original work published 1975.)

Le Guin, U. (1989). *Dancing at the edge of the world*. Grove.

Lule, J. (2001). *Daily news, eternal stories*. Guilford Press.

Moore, T. (1992). *Care of the soul*. HarperCollins.

Nelson, E. & Delmedico, A. (2023). When left hands touch: Shadow vows and Jung's quaternity. *Journal of Analytical Psychology*, 68(1), 48–70. https://doi.org/10.1111/1468-5922.12882.

Neumann, E. (1990). *Depth psychology and a new ethic* (E. Rolfe, Trans.). Shambala. (Original work published 1969.)

Otto, R. (1936). *The idea of the holy*. Oxford University Press.

Rilke, R. M. (1975). *Rilke on love and other difficulties* (J. Mood, Trans.). W. W. Norton & Co.

Schore, A. (2012). *The science of the art of psychotherapy*. W. W. Norton & Co.

Siegal, D. (2012). *The pocket guide to interpersonal neurobiology*. W. W. Norton & Co.

Solfvin, J. (1989). The healing relationship. In R. Carlson & B. Shield (Eds.), *Healers on healing* (pp. 100–103). Tarcher/Putnam.

Tacey, D. (2012). *The Jung reader*. Routledge.

van der Kolk, B. (2015). *The body keeps the score*. Penguin.

von Franz, M.-L. (1970). *An introduction to the interpretation of fairy tales*. Spring Publications.

Zimmer, C. (2004). *Soul made flesh*. Free Press.

Chapter 2

Couples and Complexes

Occasionally, everyone experiences the feeling of being out of sorts, or in the grips of something, or being beside themselves. When we see others in this frame of mind, we wonder what has gotten into them. When it is happening to us, we seemingly go on autopilot and suddenly feel taken over by something that is temporarily stronger than us. In a sense, we are temporarily out of control of ourselves and sometimes find ourselves saying or doing things we later regret. We do not just lose our temper; we lose our *tempering*. Early in his career, Jung studied this phenomenon and described this out-of-control feeling as the activation of a *complex*.[1]

When couples argue and fight in the consulting room, the felt sense of the intensely saturated quality of the atmosphere can be overwhelming for many therapists. In these instances, the psychological complexes that Jung so closely studied become activated and are usually responsible for much of the animosity on display. Otherwise, partners would be able to calmly sit with one another and discuss hard things with mutual support and empathy. But the roots of complexes run deep and remain particularly damaging and destructive in relationships unless partners become much more conscious of them. Understanding the nature of complexes helps equip therapists and couples with ways of working with these energies when they arise.

Complexes were so central to Jung's thinking that he originally called the whole of his psychology "complex psychology" before later renaming it "analytical psychology."[2] While Jung did not codify an approach to working with couples and their complexes, the imago relationship therapy formulated by Harville Hendrix and Helen Hunt is a contemporary approach that helps couples sort their parental complexes.[3] Sue Johnson's emotionally focused therapy is also rooted in work with complexes.[4] Whether naming them complexes or not, virtually all other types of therapy have conceptual frameworks to describe these moments of madness that get amplified in relationships. Complexes underpin enactments, transference, projective identification, acting out, acting in, repetition compulsions, trauma responses, dissociations, the paranoid-schizoid position, and fugue states. Any awareness that clinicians, regardless of their

DOI: 10.4324/9781032688008-3

orientation, can bring to these unconscious forces and any effort to help clarify and work with them is central to effective couples therapy.

Jung's Discovery of Complexes

Jung discovered the existence of complexes early in his career while conducting experiments using the Word Association Test (WAT) during his tenure at the Burghölzli Clinic in Zürich from 1900–1909.[5] Jung's refinements to the WAT helped it become known as the first psychological projective test.[6] The WAT is administered by reading a list of 100 words to test subjects.[7] Upon hearing each word, subjects are instructed to say the first word that comes to mind as quickly as possible. The list of words is then reread, and subjects are asked to recall their responses to each word from the first round.[8] Observers record responses and the time it takes to respond to each word. Jung also invented a variation on a galvanometer to measure minute changes in the skin's electrical conductivity, breathing, pulse rate, and perspiration.[9] In effect, he was able to measure what words made people hot under the collar, even if they were calm in outward appearance.

Jung observed and documented the widely varying responses and reactions to the Word Association Test.[10] Depending upon the individual's personal and collective history, each word can trigger a variety of responses and produce sudden variations in respiration and changes in the skin's electrical conductivity. While the test is deceptively simple, time and again, Jung found that just saying the first word that comes to mind as quickly as possible is exceedingly difficult. The stimulus words used in the test "almost without exception conjure up its corresponding situation."[11] Unusual responses or reactions indicate areas in the mind where someone is "inadequately adapted to reality."[12] Universally, no one reacts quickly and smoothly to all one hundred words. For some, certain words produce delayed reaction times or disturbances such as silence or speaking many words. Test subjects, laboring over efforts to respond, can begin to take some words personally—as if they are being questioned. Some subjects react emotionally by getting angry, agitated, dissociated, defensive, or sad. Sometimes, one of the stimulus words from one part of the test is unconsciously repeated aloud in other parts of the test.

Jung found that these responses resulted from the activation of "special psychic contents."[13] Often rooted in trauma, he called these small split-off fragments of personality an *emotionally laden complex*.[14] For couples therapists, the emotional core at the heart of complexes presents the greatest of challenges.

The Complex Defined

Jung defines complexes as "a collection of various ideas, held together by an emotional tone common to all."[15] At first blush, this is easy for therapists to understand and accept. However, Jung also observed that complexes are *autonomous* in nature. That is, they have a life of their own in the psyche. And therein lies the problem for our postmodern minds. It can be an assault on the therapist's ego to accept that they are relatively powerless in the face of an autonomous activated complex, whether it be a patient's, the couple's, or their own. It is difficult to let this truth penetrate the mind and open more fully to the possibility of helplessness when in the presence of an activated complex. A simple distinction between feelings and emotions may be useful: "We possess our feelings, but we are possessed by our emotions."[16] Jung adds, "Emotions are not 'made,' or willfully produced, in and by consciousness. Instead, they appear suddenly, leaping up from an unconscious region."[17]

Jung describes the felt sense of complexes in a variety of ways. Regarding their autonomy, Jung says, "everyone knows nowadays that people 'have complexes.' What is not so well known ... is that complexes can *have us*."[18] "An active complex puts us momentarily under a state of duress, of compulsive thinking and acting, for which under certain conditions the only appropriate term would be the judicial concept of diminished responsibility."[19] This is known offhandedly by the phrase *the devil made me do it*. Regarding their repetitive nature, Jung observes that "the complex can usually be suppressed with an effort of will, but not argued out of existence, and at the first suitable opportunity it reappears *in all its original strength* [emphasis added]."[20]

Using a scientific metaphor, Jung says that a complex's "intensity or activity curve has a wavelike character, with a 'wave-length' of hours, days, or weeks."[21] Therapists know this empirically when partners report having to take a few hours or days to calm down in the aftermath of a fight or recover from a change in mood. Jung adds, "Complexes are in fact 'splinter psyches.' The aetiology of their origin is frequently a so-called trauma, an emotional shock or some such thing, that splits off a bit of the psyche."[22] Medically, "one could best compare them with infections or with malign tumours, both of which arise without the least assistance from the conscious mind."[23]

From a spiritual perspective, Jung says, "in the Middle Ages it [the complex] went by another name: it was called possession."[24] Regarding the impact of complexes on domestic life, Jung notes, "only when you have seen whole families destroyed by them, morally and physically, and the unexampled tragedy and hopeless misery that follow in their train, do you feel the full impact of the reality of complexes."[25] Therapists know only too well the deep physical and psychological wounding from the violence that occurs when someone gets out of control.

Following Jung, over the years, a chorus of analytic therapists have further amplified the impact of complexes on intrapsychic life and relationships. The following is a brief litany:

James Hollis says that complexes "rob energy from our conscious life, oblige us to serve historic patterns rather than be in the present with all choices open, and bind us, like the mythic Ixion, to the wheel of repetition."[26] He adds, "normally we do not know we are acting out of a complex because when one is activated it has the power to take over consciousness," and we do not recognize them until "after the fact, after they have done damage."[27]

Joan Corrie says complexes "are independent of each other—little autonomous free lances, pathological units. Such complexes are the cause of obsessions, compulsions, and phobias."[28]

Murray Stein notes that when caught in a complex, "there is the depressing knowledge that one has been here many times before, has reacted in just this way on many occasions, and yet is utterly helpless to refrain from doing the same thing again this time."[29]

Robert Johnson warns, "we only know about them through the havoc they wreak in our lives and emotions."[30]

Donald Kalsched says, "complexes constitute the 'persons' of our dreams, the 'voices' in our head, the visionary figures that appear at times of stress, the 'secondary personalities' of neurosis, the daimons, ghosts and spirits that haunt or hallow the so-called primitive mind."[31]

Polly Young-Eisendrath describes the experience of being in a complex as "*just like* being in a hypnotic trance. We snap into and can snap out of it, but while we are in it we are 'elsewhere.'" She adds, "better not to go in at all. Often we do not have enough awareness to step aside and simply take note of what Otherness is arising."[32]

Psychoanalytically, Barbara Sullivan likens complexes to both Bion's notion of undigested beta elements stuck in "emotional limbo" and Winnicott's "memorized" experiences, which have been preserved in their "raw, unthinkable form in the depths of the psyche."[33]

James Hillman best summarizes the totality of the felt sense of being in the throes of an activated complex:

> Experienced *figuratively*, the complex is a personality with feelings, motivations, and memories. Experienced *somatically*, the complex is a change in heart-rate, skin-color, sphincter control, genital tumescence, breathing, sweating, etc. Experienced *energetically*, the complex is a dynamic core, accumulating ever new particles to it, like a magnet, or coalescing with other atomic units, like a molecule. It produces tension, compulsions, charged situations, transformations, attractions, repulsions. Experienced *pathologically*, the complex is an open sore that picks up every bug in the neighborhood (suggestibility), a psychic cancer growing autonomously, or a panic button, or an over-valued idea.[34]

Therapists and couples face two challenges: noticing when a complex is activated and minimizing the relational damage they may cause. The best way to notice complexes and manage through them is by trying to increase self-awareness when one is in such a state and giving voice to the agitation and misery felt in its presence. Complexes manifest in various ways, with different intensities and durations. Being aware and tracking them can reduce suffering and lessen their impact on relationships.

Jung realized the ego itself is a complex, an agglomeration of associations that comes to form what we think of as "us."[35] This is hard to fathom because we are so identified with it.[36] Psychological wholeness, then, can be considered a multiplicity consisting of ego consciousness and an unconscious replete with various and sundry autonomous complexes. There is a natural ongoing competition for control of one's thoughts, emotions, speech, behavior, and moods between the ego and unconscious complexes. Many complexes are firmly formed in early childhood, long before the ego has fully developed.[37] The ego complex functions largely unaware of these mini personalities, which are lying dormant in the unconscious waiting for opportunities for conscious expression. When one of them overtakes the ego, the ego tries to regain control and banish the scoundrel that has made us do or say something we wish we had not. Until the ego reseats itself, the psyche must contend with an uneasy sense of general malaise.

Individuals and couples live under the sway of all sorts of positive and negative complexes that often exert powerful and sometimes lifelong influences on behavior and beliefs. Here are but a few examples of the types of complexes that we can have (or that can have *us*): guilt complex, power complex, victim complex, work complex, mother or father complex, inferiority complex, savior complex, orphan complex, money complex, ego complex, duty complex, birth order complex, golden child complex, and scapegoat complex.

Complexes in Relationship

Because complexes typically operate outside of awareness, Jung cautions that they are "by no means approved by the patient, who even tries in every way to deny, or at least to weaken" their existence.[38] He stresses the importance of helping patients bring some awareness and acceptance of these "repressed" complexes, but that one must "proceed with corresponding care and tact."[39] Therapists attempt to weather the storms of the couple's activated complexes, as well as their own, and to fight, if possible, to keep their minds grounded in a stance of perpetual curiosity. This can be done by noticing and naming, with the couple, the minute changes in the emotional micro-climates of the intra- and interpsychic spaces. Therapists can also wonder aloud about their own internal reactions as they experience the couple. Instead of escaping the moment with flights to judgment, technique, or theory, therapists can strive to hold a clinical stance reminiscent of Bion's not-knowing position[40] and remain in Bachelard's cultivated state of reverie[41] while inviting couples to do the same. "Curiouser and curiouser!" as Alice reminds us.[42] But when complexes are activated, the psychological field of vision narrows, and curiosity is lost.

Much has been written about the role of the unconscious in the selection of partners, but most couples only begin to consider these more subtle forces when relationships become problematic. Lionel Corbett says, "the complex makes us look for someone who will allow us to behave in particular, auto-matic ways."[43] This initial freedom is liberating, but it eventually becomes torturous for many couples. These are the complexes that require treatment when couples enter therapy. They can be identified by asking partners what most attracted them to each other and, importantly, what is now driving them crazy about one another and how the two may be related.

While the therapist is not privy to a couple's long history of verbal and nonverbal conscious and unconscious communications (and patterns of com-munication), complexes can be recognized in sessions when the words or body language couples use with (and against) one another feel loaded. Complexes express themselves in the emotional intensity, whether hot or cold, in the room. On their best clinical behavior, some couples may reveal only the tips of the icebergs, knowing full well that so much more lies below. Therapists can slow things down with couples and inquire about the depths of what is being implied or hinted at with their verbal utterances and non-verbal communications.

By the time couples come for treatment, they have likely encountered at least one complex, the intensity of which scares or baffles them. They resort to therapy only after having tried to ignore it or work it out on their own, either privately or together, only to have the complex(es) continue to have full sway whenever activated. Therapists will also know complexes are at the root of a couple's problems when they describe their issues as a *repeating pattern*. It is often the fight they have been having for years in some form or fashion: How one partner drives, how another does not clean up after themselves, how one partner expects sex, how another always feels belittled or used. No matter what they have tried, they report ending up in the same old types of fights or conflicts and doing and saying the same old things over and over again. Hopes rise on promises of change and are dashed again each time the pattern repeats. Couples arrive for psychotherapy with a degree of despair and pessi-mism given the often years of futile attempts at improvement. They are late in getting to therapy, and years of infighting have only served to strengthen the unconscious power of their complexes.

Working with Couples and Complexes

Teasing apart which complexes are at play in a couple's conflicts and which ones belong to whom requires a detailed individual history-taking of both partners. Stein emphasizes that therapists take considerable time "tracing the history of various complexes from infancy to the present and becoming aware of how they have affected ego-consciousness in the past and continue to do so in the present."[44] When the current affect from activated complexes can be linked to their sources in early childhood wounding, the complexes begin to lose their powerful ability to disrupt and cloud the mind and allow for more intrapsychic containment. Awareness of complexes is akin to storm tracking. It is one thing to suffer while unconsciously in the grips of a complex. It is an altogether different experience to feel the first little change in emotional climate as a complex begins to activate, then track its growing intensity, experience its full force, and then observe its waning. For couples, this means letting partners know when the intensity of the internal storms are being upgraded or downgraded while taking precautions whenever possible to mitigate relational damage. Therapists can track these storms with couples in session and give voice to the felt sense in the room, which allows partners to learn how to describe their internal disturbances.

Young-Eisendrath advises that, if tolerable, these in-depth individual interviews should be conducted in the other partner's presence.[45] Not only does the interview process create an opportunity for mutual empathy about past wounding, but each partner can also practice undefended active listening without formulating responses. Further, if the interview is disturbing, therapists can observe that partner's ability to tend their own internal discomfort. After each history-taking, thoroughly processing the experience with the couple usually yields insights for them about how they listen (or do not listen) to each other and how what they hear affects them. Having the therapist mediate and reframe these conversations is essential in raising complexes to consciousness for partners in relationship. Young-Eisendrath further advises that therapists regularly remind couples that their communications with one another, especially in the presence of anxiety, stress, or conflict, are often saturated with nonrational, unconscious, complexed material. The couple is, in fact, in a stormy psychic field, though neither partner can slow down long enough to identify the changes in the atmosphere between them. Because of the strength of complexes, when one or both partners are caught in one, attempts to rationally talk them out of it is futile. Instead, therapists attuned to these moment-by-moment changes in emotional climate have an ideal vantage point and the license to slow interactions, name the changes, and investigate their roots.

Marion Woodman reminds, "when the body is holding the complex, it then becomes our most immediate access to the problem."[46] Therapists need only notice and ask about sudden changes in body position, degree of eye contact, head movement, guttural utterances, or stonewalling silences to help partners become more conscious of the strength of their complexes and help track their activation and origins. In sessions, one partner will often activate a complex (i.e., push a button) in the other to show a therapist what they have been dealing with. These overt reactions by one partner can cause the therapist to align with the other, sometimes unconsciously. However, in the interest of psychic balancing, therapists, while recognizing the overtly activated complex, can also remain curious about other complexes lying out of plain sight. Enactments do not happen in psychic vacuums, and exploring the depth of a complex for one partner often leads to an activated complex in the other. For example, if one partner is dominated by a hero complex, it may activate their partner's victim or child complex since these roles can function as a complement or counterpart to the hero.

Robert Johnson invokes the biblical allegory of the Walls of Jericho when working with complexes. He reminds therapists that sometimes many therapeutic trips around and around the impenetrable city (the complex) are required to bring any degree of consciousness to them.[47] Esther Harding notes that helping couples give voice to these emotionally laden complexes allows the relationship to tolerate more frankness and honesty. She warns that trying to suppress the fires of activated complexes is an attempt at "purchasing present peace at the cost of inevitable and increasing estrangement."[48] Each time one partner can hold and contain more of their own complex(es) and allow the other to do the same while both update one another on their internal weather, it strengthens a bond based upon intimate honesty. Ultimately, Harding says, the awareness of complexes becomes an "increased area of really worked-out understanding which nothing can destroy."[49]

Andrew Samuels notes that "sometimes we experience the content of a complex only in projection."[50] An indication of these projections occurs when the Gottmans' four horsemen (criticism, contempt, defensiveness, and stonewalling) are galloping roughshod through relationships.[51] Partners unable to tolerate emotional insight or self-assessment must unconsciously evacuate their inner disturbance(s) onto and into the other, making them the de facto reason for all misery.

James Hollis prescribes a three-pronged approach to working with complexes: Bring more awareness to them, actively dialogue with them, and watch them as they affect your life.[52] Hollis cautions to "never underestimate the power of these splinter personalities" because they "reassert themselves in ever-new form, with many disguises, amid shifting settings" arguing, "this is why we have a tendency to repeat our parent's marriage, or remain defined by it as we seek to do the opposite."[53] Assisting couples in more fully fleshing out their early recollections of family life will help them understand why some ways of being together carry so much charge or pressure.

To illuminate complexes when couples complain about their relationship, therapists can inquire, *Do these complaints feel familiar somehow? What do they remind you of in other parts of your life? Is there a pattern here? If you let your mind float back to earlier times, what comes to mind?* These types of questions kindle the partners' psyches. They invite the couple to do the hard work of making the uncomfortable and unconscious past a little more conscious and making connections between the current relational situation and its roots. With even a little empathy for each other, this subtle degree of separation and broader context can depersonalize things just enough to help partners remain connected even under such duress.

Therapists will also notice complexes at work when partners describe or enact unsavory behavior while the person acts out (or acts in) and defensively voices all manner of ready-made rationalizations for their behavior.[54] The age-old justification *See what you made me do* usually indicates someone operating under the influence of an autonomous complex. Therapists can bring therapeutic curiosity to those exchanges by asking, *Did they really make you do it? How is it that you lost control over yourself? What was happening inside you at that moment when you did what you did? Were you aware that you were losing control of yourself? Did it feel like you were powerless to stop it?* Without excusing the behavior, therapists can reframe the felt sense of the loss of control as a sign of at least one complex at work by probing further with questions from the paragraph above. A detailed exploration of the felt sense of the experience can generate considerable discomfort or agitation. However, change occurs as "the heretofore unconscious complex and the 'I' of ego are experienced concurrently as different energy states."[55] It is an active exercise in distress tolerance, and the therapist can acknowledge the tremendous psychic effort needed to hold *both* in the mind, together, simultaneously, without acting out (or in).

The therapist should also question the partner pushing the other's buttons with a similar set of questions: *How do you imagine what you were saying or doing (or not saying or doing) was affecting your partner? Could you stop yourself from doing it in the moment? What was making you do it? What was going on inside of you at that moment?* And, importantly, *What did this behavior remind you of in other or earlier areas of your life?* As couples become more aware of their complexes, partners may still come to sessions reporting similar conflicts. Now, however, the disputes are recounted with a degree of insight about themselves and the deeper emotional forces that had them in their grips. This is very hard but very good psychological work, indeed. If the reports of conflict remain as charged as before, then more trips around Johnson's proverbial Walls of Jericho will be needed.

The level of detail in the inquiries described above also helps partners differentiate. With minute attention to the external action between the couple and their internal waves of emotion, a degree of psychic separation naturally begins to occur. Each partner starts attending to what is happening inside themselves instead of focusing on the other person; they gain the ability to sort what belongs psychically to whom. (This theme is amplified again in Chapter 6 with the alchemical process of *separatio*.)

Much has been made, and rightfully so, of Martin Buber's *I–Thou* relationship.[56] In doing the work of careful separation of complexed psychic contents, Jungian analyst Mario Jacoby notes that the process is evocative of Buber's notion of an *I–It* relationship.[57] That is, one begins to have an internal degree of separation and vantage point from which to observe *It*, the full force of one's complex (or the partner's complex), while remaining separate from *It*. With this psychic achievement, one can admit, *I can see that I'm suffering or wanting to act out* instead of simply suffering or acting out. Only now are these complexes made more conscious so that they "can be corrected and transformed."[58] Going forward, this allows for the mitigation of all manner of intra-psychic and relational damage. After partners have worked through enough of their own *I–It* relationships, couples can finally enter into less contentious *I–Thou* ones.

Barbara Hannah, an analyst who studied with Jung for over twenty years, emphasizes acceptance: "Once we have realized that we are not the king in our psyche, not the master in our own house, we are—paradoxically enough—in a much stronger position."[59] Accepting this reality expands consciousness and the ability to hold more of one's own and another person's complexity. Once partners realize that they can be in the grips of something, they can feel more empathy for each other in such a state and see one another in an entirely different light. Instead of personalizing everything, they now have a degree of separation that, while not excusing behavior, allows for some grace—if they are storm tracking with one another in real-time and processing their mutual experiences afterward when working egos become available again. With this increased awareness, couples begin to limit damage, both gross and subtle, to one another and themselves.

Jungian analyst James Hall explores the bi-polar nature of complexes.[60] One part of a complex can overtake the ego, while another part is projected onto someone or something else. In couples work, that projected out part could attach itself to a partner, the marriage, a child or children, parents or in-laws, or sex, to name just a few. Efforts to de-potentiate these external figures again invite partners caught in their complexes to contain more of their affect. Holding both poles allows the psyche to work with the fullness of the complex. Partners can then take more responsibility for their own rage or despair instead of evacuating it out upon others. Working that external pole of the complex with individuals and couples after affairs, or in the drought of sexless relationships, or through separations and divorces can ultimately produce an easing of inner psychological suffering. While not eliminating the complex, it does allow for greater containment, insight, and sometimes less suffering and for shorter periods.

For couples who develop some awareness as their complexes activate, self-containment, not suppression, increasingly becomes the order of the day. Instead of acting out, partners provide cues to each other about the often dramatic shifts in their emotional climates. There are regular updates over the hours or days until complexes subside. Therapists can assist in creating the space and language to allow partners to fully experience their complexes while fostering awareness, gentleness, and mutual protection. As distress tolerance increases, couples also learn to stop pressuring one another to get over it as quickly as possible. They also quit trying to fix it or one another. Patience emerges as they learn to be with, accompany, and witness their partner. When storms hit, psychic space is now available to hunker down and ride out the weather, alone *and* together.

While this chapter has focused primarily on the insidious nature of complexes as they interfere in the lives of couples, it is important to note that positive complexes are equally as powerful and influential. Positive complexes include one's emotionally laden and affirming experiences of belonging such as allegiance to an *alma mater*, a cause, or even one's chosen therapeutic modality. Accounting for their ubiquity, Jung concludes "that autonomous complexes are among the normal phenomena of life and that they make up the structure of the unconscious."[61] He normalizes their existence, whether positive, negative, or neutral.

When working with couples, normalizing the existence and staying power of complexes, both positive and negative, helps them reconsider demands for instant change and relinquish pleas to *just get over it, finally, so we can put it behind us.* Couples who become more aware of these ubiquitous complexes now know that it is not a question of if but when and for how long each will be in the grips of something. They begin to understand that anything can trigger a complex: a look, a non-look, the holidays, a scene from a movie, a reverie in the shower, a visit with family, a song, a smell, just to name a few. Couples attune by asking and tending whatever is arising and receding in their psyches, knowing now that each is responsible for tracking their own emotional weather. They notice and share to the degree that awareness allows, creating much-needed psychic space between them as well as emotional intimacy. A sense of easefulness, lightheartedness, and even playfulness often returns.

With such conscious and unconscious pressure on therapists to limit sessions and ease couples' immediate tensions, they often ignore these underlying activated complexes—the Rosetta Stone for relational discord. Clinicians can recast a couple's symptoms as complexes with emotional cores crying out for attention instead of problems to be adjudicated and banished. "A symptom develops not 'because of' prior history, but 'in order to' express a piece of psyche or accomplish a purpose. The clinical question is not reductive, but synthetic."[62] Instead of worrying, *How can I quickly lessen a couple's symptoms?*, curious therapists wonder and ask, *What is this symptom for? What is all this fighting really about? What purpose is it serving in the relationship? What deeper truth is this misery trying to express about one or both partners or their relationship? What earlier wounding might be calling out for more attention?* To explore these questions, clinicians must develop an expanded holding capacity. They must not only tolerate the presence of an activated complex, but also be able to turn toward the full force of it and seek its roots so that everyone can become more conscious of it. Only then does the power of the complex diminish, freeing partners from its grips. Therapists model with couples how to explore, witness, and be with one another through these periods of activation.

Couples Therapists and Their Complexes

Couples therapy requires engaging, if possible, with live complexes while they are flourishing in the consulting room. Tavistock Institute of Marital Studies' James Fisher remarks, "the intense acting out and acting in sweep the therapists up as if they had awakened to find themselves in someone else's nightmare."[63] Being caught up in the couple's complex(es) activates the dormant complexes in the mind and body of the attuned couples therapist. This presents a tremendous psychological challenge for any therapist.

Some therapists with limited experience working with couples report feeling shocked or overwhelmed by the intensity of live interactions, which typically far exceeds that of individual sessions.[64] Once they get some experience with couples therapy, most have a strong preference: they either love it or hate it. When asked how they responded when they were little to their parents fighting, the ones who hate it often report that they ran and hid, while those who love it recount running into the fray and getting between parents trying to break it up.

Complexes are activated in both types of therapists. For those who fled the primal parental scene, their work is to be with their complexed material and work through it as they sit uncomfortably now as an adult through charged sessions with others. It takes tremendous courage and often a heroic effort to sit in one's activated complex(es) and to become more conscious of them and their effects on the body and the mind so that their impact can lessen over time. Therapists who love couples therapy and played referee and peacemaker as a child have to deal with a different type of activated complex. They must resist the urge to jump in too quickly, take over, and put everyone on ice. There is no psychological growth for couples with a peace-at-all-costs approach.

As trauma-informed therapists may surmise, there is also a third kind of therapist who reports simply freezing in sessions when couples start fighting. They report not fleeing or fighting, but simply watching as couples fight on, sometimes for entire sessions, unable to speak or even bring sessions to an end on time. A third type of complex is at work, which requires the courage to stand in while trying to find one's adult voice *and* manage frightened and paralyzed younger inner selves. The complexed responses (or lack thereof) of therapists most often have their roots in their own unresolved trauma. Additional psychological work is indicated for therapists dealing with their complexes activated by the types of intense therapeutic encounters found in couples therapy. Jung warns:

> No investigator [or therapist], however unprejudiced and objective he is, can afford to disregard his own complexes, for they enjoy the same autonomy as those of other people. As a matter of fact, they *cannot* disregard them because they do not disregard *him*.[65]

Therefore, therapists can abandon the illusion of therapeutic neutrality and make peace with the fact that their complexes cannot be ignored or bracketed out. Complexes are the very lens(es) through which we take in the world. As surely as couples are caught in their complexes, therapists are caught in their own. How else can one explain the wide variety of countertransferences, intrapsychic reactions, enactments, and other affects experienced by therapists hour over therapeutic hour, or just the mood shifts when clinical material from the day still reverberates?

Conclusion

Perhaps the best advice when caught in a complex is the same counter-intuitive advice given to swimmers when caught in a rip tide: *Relax, and don't fight it. The currents pulling on you are much stronger than you know. Once you get your bearings, try to swim parallel to the shore until you are out of the current. Then, slowly make your way back to shore at an angle.* Therapists can help couples recognize when one or both partners are caught in a complex. Learning to communicate about it in real-time is challenging. Self-care is paramount during those times. Couples can learn how to let each other know when they are caught in a complex, provide each other with ample supportive space to sort out what is happening, and then welcome their return as they make their way back to the shore of the relationship.

In a broader sense, much of the world's nonrational behavior can be accounted for by utilizing Jung's concept of emotionally toned autonomous complexes, both positive and negative, whether individual, cultural, or collective.[66] Closer to home, complexes are constantly emerging and subsiding within and between us. Whether aware of it or not, we are all usually in the grips of something. It is only a matter of degree. Just as we cannot banish the weather, we cannot banish complexes: we live with them and, with skill and attention, become adept storm-trackers.

Notes

1 Jung 1973.
2 Sedgwick 2001, p. 30.
3 Hendrix & Hunt 2021.
4 Johnson 2019.
5 Ellenberger 1970.
6 Klopfer et al. 1955. According to Ellenberger (1970), Jung's improvements to the WAT prompted the development of other projective tests including the Rorschach. It is also the basis for the lie detector test.
7 During its evolution, the Word Association Test had as many as 400 words. Jung finally settled on following 100: head, green, water, to sing, death, long, ship, to pay, window, friendly, table, to ask, cold, stem, to dance, village, lake, sick, pride, to cook, ink, angry, needle, to swim, journey, blue, lamp, to sin, bread, rich, tree, to prick, pity, yellow, mountain, to die, salt, new, custom, to

pray, money, stupid, exercise-book, to despise, finder, dear, bird, to fall, book, unjust, frog, to part, hunger, white, child, to pay attention, pencil, sad, plum, to marry, house, darling, glass, to quarrel, fur, big, carrot, to paint, part, old, flower, to beat, box, wild, family, to wash, cow, friend, happiness, lie, deportment, narrow, brother, to fear, stork, false, anxiety, to kiss, bride, pure, door, to choose, hay, contended, ridicule, to sleep, month, nice, woman, to abuse (Jung 1909).

8   Jung 1973.
9   Bair 2003.
10   Jung 1973.
11   Jung 1973, para. 944.
12   Jung 1973, para. 944.
13   Jung 1911, para. 1351.
14   Along with the groundbreaking work of Ferenczi (1955), Janet (2019[1925]), and Freud (1914), Jung's (1973) discovery of complexes also forms the foundations of modern trauma theory (Gazzaniga 1998; Tresan 1996; Van der Kolk 2014). While the focus of this book is not trauma *per se*, one can consider, for the sake of couples therapy, that the intensely saturated conflictual interactions between partners are activated complexes echoing the psyche's long-forgotten and embedded traumatic experiences.
15   Jung 1911, para. 1350.
16   Harms 1950, p. 153.
17   Jung 1950, p. 10.
18   Jung 1934, para. 200.
19   Jung 1934, para. 200.
20   Jung 1934, para. 201.
21   Jung 1934, para. 201
22   Jung 1934, para. 204.
23   Jung 1934, para. 209.
24   Jung 1934, para. 204.
25   Jung 1934, para. 209.
26   Hollis 2005, pp. 96–97.
27   Hollis 2005, p. 118.
28   Corrie 2015[1927], p. 64.
29   Stein 1998, p. 43.
30   Johnson 1986, p. 204.
31   Kalsched 1996, p. 90.
32   Young-Eisendrath 1993, p. 73.
33   Sullivan 2010, p. 73.
34   Hillman 1974 pp. 190–191.
35   Jung 1911, para. 1352.
36   Those with more than one identity (dissociative identity disorder) have at least one other ego-like complex, each acting autonomously and coming to the forefront when sufficiently activated.
37   Van Eenwyk 1997.
38   Jung 1911, para. 1351.
39   Jung 1911, para. 1351.
40   Bion 1967.
41   Bachelard 1960.
42   Carol 1992[1865], p. 21.
43   Corbett 2007, p. 80.
44   Stein 1995, p. 43.

45 Young-Eisendrath 1984. To help therapists bring couples complexes to light, Young-Eisendrath also includes a Psychosexual Assessment and Developmental Assessment in Context in the Appendix of this exceptional work.
46 Woodman 1980, p. 61.
47 Johnson 1986.
48 Harding 1970, p. 143.
49 Harding 1970, p. 143.
50 Samuels 1985, p. 48.
51 Gottman & Gottman 2015.
52 Hollis 2005.
53 Hollis 2005, p. 97.
54 Hollis 2005.
55 Vesey-McGrew 2010, p. 17.
56 Buber 2010[1923].
57 Jacoby 1984.
58 Jacobi 1959, p. 11.
59 Hannah 1976, p. 109.
60 Hall 1989.
61 Jung 1934, para. 218.
62 Salmon 1997, p, 62.
63 Fisher 2019, p. 75.
64 Though born of necessity in the COVID pandemic, it is nevertheless interesting to note the rapid and wide acceptance, popularity, and *continued* practice of therapy via screens, phones, and even texting. Perhaps clinicians, though unwilling to admit it, are relieved to get some distance, albeit virtual, from the intensity of co-created live psychic space where activated complexes wreak havoc on all psyches in the consulting room.
65 Jung 1934, para. 213.
66 Though beyond the scope of this introduction, *The Cultural Complex* (Singer & Kimbles 2004) collects essays exploring the impact of complexes on a variety of contemporary and historical events.

References

Bachelard, G. (1960). *The poetics of reverie*. Beacon Press.
Bair, D. (2003). *Jung: A biography*. Back Bay Books.
Bion, W. (1967). Notes on memory and desire. *The Psychoanalytic Forum*, 2(3), 271–280.
Buber, M. (2010). *I and thou* (R. G. Smith, Trans.). Martino Publishing. (Original work published 1923.)
Carol, L. (1992). *Alice's adventures in wonderland*. Knopf. (Original work published 1865.)
Corbett, L. (2007). *Psyche and the sacred*. Spring Journal Books.
Corrie, J. (2015). *ABC of Jung's psychology*. Routledge. (Original work published 1927.)
Ellenberger, H. (1970). *The discovery of the unconscious*. Basic Books.
Ferenczi, S. (1955). *Final contributions to the problems & methods of psycho-analysis* (E. Mosbacher and others, Trans.) (M. Balint, Ed.). Basic Books.
Fisher, J. V. (2019). *The uninvited guest*. Routledge.
Freud, S. (1914). Remembering, repeating, and working-through. *SE* XII.
Gazzaniga, M. S. (1998). *The mind's past*. University of California Press.
Gottman, J. S., & Gottman, J. M. (2015). *10 Principles for doing effective couples therapy*. Norton.

Hall, J. A. (1989). *Hypnosis: A Jungian perspective.* Guilford Press.

Hannah, B. (1976). *Jung: His life and work.* G. P. Putnam's Sons.

Harding, M. E. (1970). *The way of all women.* Shambhala.

Harms, E. (1950). A differential concept of feelings and emotions. In M. L. Reymert (Ed.), *Feelings and emotions* (pp. 147–157). McGraw-Hill Book Company.

Hendrix, H., & Hunt, H. L. (2021). *Imago relationship therapy.* Norton.

Hillman, J. (1974). Archetypal theory. In *Loose ends* (pp. 170–195). Spring Publications.

Hollis, J. (2005). *Finding meaning in the second half of life.* Gotham Books.

Jacobi, J. (1959). *Complex/archetype/symbol in the psychology of C. G. Jung.* Princeton University Press.

Jacoby, M. (1984). *The analytic encounter.* Inner City Books.

Janet, P. (2019). *Psychological healing* (Vols. I & II). Martino Fine Books. (Original work published 1925.)

Johnson, R. A. (1986). *Inner work.* HarperOne.

Johnson, S. M. (2019). *Attachment theory in practice.* Guilford Press.

Jung, C. G. (1909). The association method. *CW* 2.

Jung, C. G.(1911). On the doctrine of the complexes. *CW* 2.

Jung, C. G.(1934). A review of complex theory. *CW* 8.

Jung, C. G.(1950). *The integration of the personality.* Routledge & Kegan Paul.

Jung, C. G.(1973). *Experimental researches. CW* 2.

Kalsched, D. (1996). *The inner world of trauma.* Routledge.

Klopfer, B., Bash, K. W., & Riklin, F. (1955). C. G. Jung and projective techniques. *Journal of Projective Techniques*, 19(3), 225–270. https://doi.org/10.1080/08853126. 1955.10380631.

Salmon, S. (1997). The creative psyche: Jung's major contributions. In P. Young-Eisendrath & T. Dawson (Eds.), *The Cambridge companion to Jung* (pp. 52–70). Cambridge University Press.

Samuels, A. (1985). *Jung and the post-Jungians.* Routledge.

Sedgwick, D. (2001). *Introduction to Jungian psychotherapy.* Routledge.

Singer, T., & Kimbles, S. L. (Eds.). (2004). *The Cultural Complex.* Routledge.

Stein, M. (1995). The aims and goal of Jungian analysis. In M. Stein (Ed.), *Jungian analysis* (2nd edn, pp. 29–49). Open Court.

Stein, M.(1998). *Jung's map of the soul.* Open Court.

Sullivan, B. S. (2010). *The mystery of analytical work.* Routledge.

Tresan, D. I. (1996). Jungian metapsychology and neurobiological theory. *Journal of Analytical Psychology*, 41, 399–436.

Van der Kolk, B. A. (2014). *The body keeps the score.* Viking.

Van Eenwyk, J. R. (1997). *Archetypes & strange attractors.* Inner City Books.

Vesey-McGrew, P. (2010). Getting on top of thought and behavior patterns. In M. Stein (Ed.), *Jungian analysis* (2nd edn, pp. 14–21). Open Court.

Woodman, M. (1980). *The owl was a baker's daughter.* Inner City Books.

Young-Eisendrath, P. (1984). *Hags and heroes.* Inner City Books.

Young-Eisendrath, P.(1993). *You're not what I expected.* William Morrow and Company.

Chapter 3

The Archetypal Basis of Coupled Life

Couples therapists are all too familiar with the metaphors partners use—their figures of speech—to describe the turmoil in their relationship. Consider: *This relationship has become an albatross around my neck. You are like an iceberg. We're ships passing in the night. You're a pig. You're like a leech sucking the life out of me. Quit treating me like a child.* Each metaphor, charged with energy, expresses an emotional truth for the suffering partner. The images at the core of the metaphors—*albatross, iceberg, ships, pig, leech, child*—naturally arise in heated conversations. They are alive with meaning, far more meaning than most people realize. A Jungian approach regards such images as the way the psyche expresses itself, the soul's own language. Clinically, images also provide therapists with a direct way to work with couples embroiled in entrenched conflict.

The intensity of the energies surrounding the images couples use to describe their frustrations often leaves therapists at a loss. Such potent images, Jung says, have an *archetypal* core,[1] making Jung's theory of archetypes, along with his complex theory, particularly relevant to couples therapists. Longstanding conflict is anchored in archetypal roles and patterns. Working with them is working at the very foundation of the couple's suffering.

When therapists can slow down and amplify an image, it kindles the minds of both partners and helps reveal the multiple and layered meanings of the image—meanings that continue to unfold over time. James Hillman, an early protégé of Jung's who became one of the co-founders of archetypal psychology says, "the depth of even the simplest image is truly fathomless."[2] Perhaps there is no such thing as a simple image when it has captivated our attention since "the more we reflect on it, the more we discover in it."[3] When therapists express curiosity about the images couples inject into therapy—usually spontaneously, simply in what they say in the moment—then they can help couples notice, value, and trust the images as inner guides for themselves and for their relationship. Image work invites deep connection to the depths of one's one being, which evolves over time, taking on (or revealing) new qualities. "This unending, embracing depth is one way that dreams [and images] show their love."[4]

DOI: 10.4324/9781032688008-4

Whereas archetypal psychology focusses its attention on the archetypal *image*—the meaningful, individual experience of the image as it presents itself here and now—Jung took pains to define the archetype as such, describing it in different ways.[5] He says archetypes are the elemental forms of the collective unconscious, which is a species memory reflecting the instinctual basis of human life and the outpourings of human culture. Archetypes are forms or patterns without content, something like the silhouette of a figure rather than a full-color drawing. Although there are countless archetypes (forms, patterns) that influence us, Jung names and explores a few prominent ones throughout his *Collected Works*: ego, shadow, anima/animus, Self, mother, father, child, trickster, hero, orphan, wise old man, wise old woman. Jung insists, "the archetype itself is empty and purely formal"[6] and remains abstract until the form is filled in, although their name and "invariable nucleus of meaning" makes them recognizable.[7] When the empty form is filled in, then we speak of an *archetypal image*.

For example, Mother is an archetype composed of all maternal qualities or attributes, both good and bad. When the pure, empty form of the archetype Mother is filled in with personal qualities drawn from decades of experience with her, then we can speak of an *archetypal image* of Mother. An experience of one's actual mother generates specific associations such as warmth or coldness, affection or neglect, and a host of other attributes. The *archetypal image* of Mother and those specific qualities will be unique to each person, powerfully influencing a couple's home life since their home will reflect early family life, for better and for worse. Another example is the Healer archetype. Its nucleus of meaning centers upon common attributes including an ethic of care, service to others, and dedication to health and wholeness. As an archetype, Healer becomes meaningful—that is, a concrete archetypal image versus an abstract idea—when it is embodied in particular people such as therapists, nurses, doctors, midwives, spiritual directors, or yoga instructors.

Jung describes archetypes as "deposits of the constantly repeated experiences of humanity."[8] The archetypal layers of the psyche are like foundational geological strata that have accumulated over a vast period of time. In a similar earthy metaphor, he compares archetypes to a dry riverbed, "an old watercourse along which the water of life has flowed for centuries, digging a deep channel for itself."[9] The more ancient the watercourse—that is, the older the archetypal pattern—the more readily the pattern will be refilled or reused. Elsewhere Jung draws from humanity's long love affair with stories, especially stories that bespeak the religious instinct and satiate our endless hunger for meaning, to explain archetypes. "The archetype is a kind of readiness to produce over and over again the same or similar mythical ideas" or literary themes.[10]

The breadth of Jung's metaphors—from earthy geographical images to mythic spiritual ones—express the full scope of archetypal influence on human experience. When an archetypal pattern is activated, it moves body, mind, and soul. As "modes of apprehension" or ways of seeing, archetypal images produce our attitudes, thoughts, beliefs, or insights.[11] As instinctual patterns of behavior—to protect, love, nurture, cooperate, compete, control, defend, and more—they motivate action, from a couple's subtlest gestures and daily habits to life-changing decisions about their future.

The archetype "always brings with it a certain influence or power" and "either exercises a numinous or a fascinating effect, or impels to action."[12] Therapists can recognize the power of archetypes by the sheer energy and conviction with which couples speak or when there is a repetitive nature to their conflicts. The repetition, which can dull a therapist's senses, is also quite meaningful. The psyches in the room are trying to bring the couple and therapist back to yet another version of the same archetypal problem by repeating it over and over in a variety of ways. Just as geologists sometimes lick rocks to help identify their composition, therapists keep getting a similar taste when the couple's discord is archetypal despite the variety of topics they fight about. Even though each fight is over something different, somehow, they feel the same.

The repetitive nature of archetypal problems in a relationship offers a clue about archetypal (valuable) images. Like a beloved animal who follows you from room to room, an archetypal image wants attention—and it will keep dogging your heels until it gets it. There is another similarity between archetypal images and companion animals, which is unsurprising since Hillman says "images are animated like an animal"[13] Archetypal images bear gifts—of insight, understanding, wisdom, and love. They "mean well for us, back us up and urge us on, understand us more deeply than we understand ourselves, expand our sensuousness and spirit, continually make up new things to give to us," which includes the "feeling of being loved."[14]

Hillman uses *archetypal* as an adjective. That is, what is *archetypal* for couples is valuable, meaningful, memorable, and generative. "By attaching 'archetypal' to an image, we ennoble or empower the image with the widest, richest, and deepest possible significance," and then we can describe it as "unfathomable, patterned, hidden, rich, prior, deep, necessary, permanent."[15] Of course, not all images possess this level of significance, just as not all moments in life are memorable. As Hillman admits, "if one can say 'so what' to an image, it is hardly archetypal."[16] Therapists working with metaphorical images help couples get to the archetypal roots of their painful, repetitive conflicts and long-standing interlocking relational patterns. They also begin to notice what is archetypal (meaningful) for them, and come to rely upon their own images, inner figures, and working metaphors as guides.

The Bipolar Nature of Archetypes

Archetypes are bipolar in nature, with one end positive and the other negative.[17] For example, the positive pole of the Mother archetype is a collection of all the welcome, nurturing attributes of motherhood, while the negative attributes of Mother collect at the other end. Therapists can recognize the two poles of an archetype in the phenomenon of *splitting*. Splitting occurs when partners are stuck in either end, the negative (bad) pole or the positive (good) pole, or when one partner projects one of the poles onto the other. By the time couples come to therapy, at least one partner has become the problem, the holder of the negative side of an archetypal pattern. Often, they are both projecting the negative archetypal pole onto the other. Sometimes, in order to protect the other, one partner will assume the role of identified problem and claim sole ownership of the negative pole. By exploring the complexity of archetypal patterns that show up in splitting, therapists can help work through the polarized either/or positions to help usher in both/and positions, helping partners reclaim the good *and* bad aspects of themselves and each other.

Therapists can help partners recognize and accept both the positive and negative poles of any archetypal constellation. For example, couples with children often struggle with the complicated feelings that come with parenting. They strive to be ideal parents, but children are demanding, often uncooperative, and exhausting. A parent trying to be good can only be good for so long, and then, despite the best of intentions, the bad side surfaces. Partners have a difficult time initially accepting the bipolar nature of parenting, whether they embody the Mother or Father archetype. If parents do not accept and normalize the existence of both poles within themselves, then the unacknowledged pole is forced into the unconscious or projected onto their partner, where it only gains power. Accepting that everyone carries the *potential* for both helps couples heal the good parent/bad parent split that can occur in families. Mothers and fathers can both be nurturers and limit setters; both can be patient and at their wit's end.

To help couples realize and accept the negative sides of their parenting archetype, therapists work to give a fuller voice to just how much their children sometimes drive them crazy. A parent fearful or unfamiliar with the intense energies at the negative pole of parenting might say, *I love my child and would do anything for them, but sometimes I get so frustrated, I want to destroy them. And then I feel so bad about having that thought that I want to destroy myself instead.* Or, *I'm so glad I became a parent and can't imagine my life without my child(ren), but sometimes it gets so bad that I wish I had never had them and sometimes even regret ever being born myself.* Both poles of the archetype are being internally experienced: the idealized good parent and the destructive bad parent. Partners are often afraid to talk about the intensity of these universally experienced negative feelings. However, helping couples speak more freely helps them metabolize the energies instead of acting them out.

As partners come to know the fullness of both poles, they can say without fear or shame and with wisdom tempered by the truth: *I aspire to be a great parent, but I also know that I have the potential to be a really bad one, just like everyone else who has ever tried to raise a child. Now, I can more easily watch myself being pulled between these two poles, moment by moment, as I parent my child.* When couples no longer deny or repress the negative pole of an archetypal pattern, but instead work it through, it is drained of its power and the need to erupt long before they ever have a chance of acting it out.

Archetypal Pairings in the Couple Relationship

Couples therapists must contend with archetypal pairings when the partners have divided roles. Some common examples include: good parent/bad parent, hero/helpless, student/teacher, angel/devil, parent/child, sensitive/stoic, optimist/pessimist, sexual/frigid, wounded/healer, fixed/broken. These pairings appear in the intense emotions, deep needs, longings, or frustrations partners express and whenever partners are stuck in a narrow range of possible ways to think or behave with each other. Therapists can use archetypal insight to recognize a couple's entrenched roles as the deep background affecting the couple's relationship.

A therapist's countertransference also yields clues about a couple's archetypal pairings. For example, distressed partners may evoke in the therapist a sense that partners are like lost and confused children desperately in need of maternal care, or spoiled children in need of scolding or discipline. In either case, the therapist feels unconsciously pressured into a parenting role, either nurturing or stern, which is a clue to the presence of a parent/child archetypal constellation at work in the couple. They can wonder aloud with the couple about each partner's experience of mothering or fathering. *When you're fighting with each other, how old you feel? I sense that you need some nurturing, is that true?* Or, *When you argue, are you hoping someone gets in trouble?* In this kind of conversation, everyone can be curious about the power that the parent/child archetypal pattern has over the relationship. Once couples recognize and explore the patterns, it expands their understanding and helps them reimagine their conflict in more complex ways—even if things do not immediately change.

Some archetypal patterns quickly emerge and recede in a couple's relationship, while others slowly emerge and recede over time. Some exert powerful influences over a lifetime. Regardless, awareness of the patterns can lessen suffering. For example, consider someone whose partner continually embodies the Hero archetype. Instead of unconsciously sliding into their usual Helpless role, they can name the action with their partner: *There you are! My hero coming to save the day again! Thanks for trying to rescue me, but I want to figure this out for myself. And wait, you don't have to leave. You can stay close and cheer me on while I get this sorted, and then we can celebrate together.*

In this exchange, the Hero still gets full credit for trying to help—which is what heroes like to do—yet they are invited to embody a different archetypal pattern of helping, that of Nurturer or Witness, which allows their partner to use their own capacity and skillfulness instead of remaining helpless. Problems that activate the Hero archetype are surprisingly common and mundane. They appear everywhere in everyday life and are easy for couples to explore. Consider the following situations: A light bulb is burnt out in the hallway. The baby's diaper needs changing. The car needs an oil change. We are out of milk. There's a spider in the bathroom. I had a fight with my boss at work. How much money do we have in our account? Did you have an orgasm? The dog needs to go out. I'm hungry.

Therapists help couples see through their struggles to the powerful inter-locking archetypal patterns. Placing day-to-day conflicts in this context gen-erates insight and encourages wonder. It even invites humor: *There you go again. You are so quick to charge into battle to save the day!* Or, *Look at you climbing up into your tower hoping someone will come and rescue you.* To increase awareness, therapists remind partners how these patterns interlock: If one partner is not always trying to be the Hero, the other will not always need rescuing. Conversely, if one partner is not always in need of saving, the other will not always be needing to play the Hero. Therapists know that it is very difficult for archetypally constellated Heroes to stop doing what they do. They either rush in to save the day, or when thwarted, they get frustrated and become angry and shut down. It sometimes takes considerable work with Heroic part-ners to help them find other ways of being that do not include just rescuing or shutting down. As the strength of the interlocking archetypal pairings lessen, couples are free to try on other less restrictive roles. Working archetypally grounds and normalizes couples' discord in humanity's timeless past. It invites partners into the future with more insight about their drama and provides much-needed psychological flexibility to help them reshape their story.

The Drama of the Couple

Therapists can discover archetypal material by using another of Jung's meta-phors: imagining a couple's relationship in theatrical terms.[18] Therapists can wonder, *Who are the interesting characters in their stories? What are they doing with and to one another? What story is wanting to be told here?* Since the psyche is always changing, always in movement, an archetypal approach invites therapists and partners to notice what is happening in the moment as dramas unfold. This week, one figure (or image or metaphor) may stand out in the way a talented actor draws an audience's attention. Next week, it may be someone or something else. Imagining a couple's interactions as theater, albeit theater of the most serious kind, invites curiosity. Therapists and cou-ples notice the soul's movement—rather than trying to fix or freeze it. As inner figures, such characters symbolize the multiple aspects of each partner's identity, including known, developed capacities and yet-to-be-known poten-tial capacities. Over time, these inner figures may come to feel like old friends or members of their own psychological family guiding them toward individuation.

Jung uses the metaphor of theater to describe working with images, yet cautions against remaining in the passive role of audience. The image "does not want merely to be watched impartially ... it wants to compel participation."[19] He adds, "if the observer understands that his own drama is being performed on this inner stage, he cannot remain indifferent to the plot and its denouement."[20] Inviting couples to deepen into their drama, therapists can ask them to actively engage with their images: *Describe what is happening here. If you were to embody the figure, what else might they want to say? What other figures are hiding in the shadows? What might they say?* The remarkable psychological impact of play is often undervalued since adults are supposed to grow out of their imagination. Yet actively working with a couple's images in the theater of their relationship is relational and participatory. "We get into the images, and the images get into us."[21]

Working with a couple's images makes it possible to "be precise in what we say about the soul of the relationship when it is full of ambiguity and mystery."[22] Therapists can amplify images anytime they arise in therapy. There is a very good chance that the couple making their first appointment has already diagnosed themselves or, more problematically, one another, which presents therapists with one of the first challenges: To peel away labels and the illusion of certainty that labels provide and shift the work to archetypal levels. Dropping into the archetypal level can be done at the outset of therapy. Rather than pressing to get through an intake, therapists can notice the metaphors couples use to describe their situation and slow down to explore the image within the metaphor. One partner might say, *Our relationship feels like it's on life support.* Listening with an archetypal ear, a therapist can ask, *Did you say, "on life support?" How long has it been on life support? What happened to it? What is the prognosis?* Turning to the other partner: *Does it feel like it's on life support to you, too?* The other partner usually has a different notion of the problem and a different metaphor. They might reply, *No, it's not dying. For me, it's more like it's dried out. Like in a desert.* The therapist notes, *So for one of you it's on life support, and for the other it's dried out, stuck in the desert.* With that, the therapist now has working metaphors that are meaningful for the couple, different images that are alive and native to their own psyches, useful indicators of how the therapy is proceeding. Often, new metaphors take the place of old ones and offer new images. A partner might say, *Oh, it's no longer on life support. But now, it's like there's a wall between us.* Noting this shift, the therapist amplifies the new image, *A wall? What kind of wall? How tall and thick is it? How do you think it got there? Where are you two in relation to it?*

Therapists welcome metaphors with an abiding curiosity, enlivening them for their own sake.[23] If the image of a wall has entered the conversation, they do not try to use it to manipulate the therapy, as in *What can I have the couple do to break down the wall?* The psyche easily recognizes attempts at manipulation, the kinds of directive therapy questions—ego-centered and goal-driven—that only serve to kill the image and shut down the work. Simple acceptance is friendlier, and it demonstrates respect for the psyche's vernacular.

Archetypal couples therapy trusts that the images emerging from a partner's deep psyche have something important to say about the relationship. Therapists can help couples regard them as a source of insight. When partners have moved out of crisis mode and attained some measure of peace with each other, therapists might do more than simply note the images that naturally arise in the work. They can invite the partners to bring one or more images of the relationship to the next session or invite the partners to collaborate in making a collage of meaningful images that express their coupled life.

Working with images "is psychology in the wider meaning of the word, a psychological activity of creative nature, in which creative fantasy is given prior place."[24] It requires adopting an attitude of hospitality, welcoming the images as Mary Watkins describes, or seeing the world by way of images, as Edward Casey explains.[25] Fundamentally, partners can learn to notice the active presence of images and their continual generosity. It is as though caring for one's soul is a joint undertaking: each partner and their important images tending soul together, each helping steer the relationship through its rocky passages with deft hands on the tiller. Over time, therapists develop archetypal eyes (to see the images and inner figures), ears (to hear the metaphors), and senses (to pick up on the energy) in the recurring patterns that keep couples stuck. They also notice the archetypal movements in their own souls, both in and out of sessions. Valuing and trusting their own images more fully, therapists also rely on them to help guide the work as well.[26]

The Couple's Mythology and Archetypal Motifs

In his research on archetypes, Jung recognized a direct connection between archetypal images and mythology.[27] Therapists know this instinctively when couples describe fairytale-like hopes and nightmarish encounters. All of us, says Jung, inherit the tendency "to form representations of mythological motifs" found in human culture, yet individual representations of these motifs, the archetypal images, "vary a great deal without losing their basic pattern."[28] For example, the Hero archetype is found in all cultures throughout time, but the motif is fleshed out in an infinite variety of ways.[29]

Attuned therapists begin to recognize archetypal motifs in couples' personal stories and hear the deeper music of their mythological background. Drawing upon mythic stories from multiple cultural traditions enriches and deepens therapeutic moments. Therapists can encourage couples to explore their inherited traditions or recall stories they loved as children. Partners might reflect upon contemporary stories they return to again and again, a novel they re-read, or movies they have seen a dozen times. Stories *are* medicine. Therapists help partners understand why their favorite stories mean so much to them. By simultaneously dwelling in the partner's personal world and the objective world of the collective unconscious, therapists attend to what is alive for couples both individually and mythically. Metaphoric resonance joins the two.

Jung insists on rooting his psychology in myth. Mythic sensibility is essential to the art of life, "the most distinguished and rarest of all the arts."[30]

> Man is not complete when he lives in a world of statistical truth. He must live in the world of his mythological truth, and that is not merely statistics. It is an expression of what he really is, and what he feels himself to be. A man without mythology is merely a product of statistics, as it were, an average phenomenon.[31]

Stories about couples are found in histories, myths, legends, poems, and fairy tales from all over the world.[32] Imaginative contemporary authors retell the tales, too, revealing their timeless themes and motifs. When therapists recognize an archetypal pattern, they connect partners to a relevant story to help them normalize and understand their struggles in a larger context.

Excursion: The *Homeric Hymn to Demeter* in the Twenty-first Century

A couple enters therapy to focus on the tension between her need for solitude and his feeling of rejection when she takes time apart for herself. (This is a common theme for couples trying to balance the need for both autonomy and intimacy.) In describing to the therapist how they met and fell in love, the woman tells a story the couple has laughed about many times. The husband, following an old-fashioned tradition, wanted to formally seek his future mother-in-law's permission to marry her daughter. At a nice restaurant over dessert, he asks. The couple is fully anticipating an enthusiastic *Yes*. Instead, her mother pauses, then says, *I'll loan her to you for a while.* Everyone moves past this startling response with awkward laughter, and the couple marries some months later.

Thinking about other stories where loyalties are in question, the therapist, who had an interest in Greek literature, recognized this motif from the *Homeric Hymn to Demeter*, the story of a powerful mother (Demeter, goddess of the Earth) whose nameless daughter is abducted into the underworld. Demeter demands the return of her daughter, but she only gets *part* of what she wants. During the winter, her daughter must live with her husband, Hades, in the underworld. In springtime, she can leave the underworld and her husband to dwell on earth. Demeter, very reluctantly, has had to *loan her daughter* to the underworld.

From the mother's perspective this is a story of loss. From the daughter's, it is quite different. She was once nameless, known only through a dependent relationship on a formidable goddess. Through her descent, she symbolically dies as the Kore (Greek for "young girl") and is reborn as Persephone, the powerful queen of the underworld. Sharing this story, or any other with similar themes that may resonate, helps amplify both the daughter's frustrations of being torn between two situations and the husband's frustrations over endless competition for attention.

When couples realize that their recurrent struggles often have archetypal or mythic underpinnings, they get to know a larger cast of characters playing a role in the drama of their relationship. Characters and patterns resurface again and again, as mentioned earlier. Like a musical motif in a symphony, they are repeated many times by different instruments with slight variations, yet all resonate with one another. Couples and therapists notice these uncanny similarities when the energies holding couples in these patterns start to feel familiar.

When working with couples, therapists may wonder about just how much influence they have over these archetypally bound interactions. The answer may appear to be *very little* because when working with inner images, change is usually subtle at first. Nonetheless, images are psychological facts for couples, and therapists can follow them closely to bring forth associated stories, ideas, intuitions, sensations, emotions, moods, and figures. The process is freeform and dream-like rather than goal-oriented. "We no longer direct our thoughts along a definite track, but let them float, sink, or rise according to their specific gravity."[33] Jung's images (float, sink, rise) suggest the fluid quality of the process. Thus, a paradox: Although intentionally aimless, this kind of thinking is psychologically productive. "Just by amplifying we do therapy ... we re-connect, remember ourselves with a wider imagination."[34] Working archetypally, therapists may also find themselves holding diagnostic labels and treatment plans more lightly. Progress may not so much be charted by numbers of sessions or improvements or setbacks couples report on, but rather it may be more authentically noted by archetypal roles loosening their grips, greater fluidity in relational patterns, and new images and energies emerging while others recede.

Archetypal material saturates couples therapy in large part because partners settle into complementary and opposing roles much as they settled into childhood patterns described in Chapter 5. Psychologically, it is easier to hold up one end of an opposing archetypal pole rather than expressing both—along with all the shades of thought and behavior in between. An image for dividing the roles between the partners is the childhood game "tug of war," in which players hold their end of the rope, dig in with their heels, and try not to let go. This image is an apt metaphor for polarized and polarizing roles in relationships where partners refuse to relinquish their opposing positions. Their split archetypal roles fix them against one another making it an interminable archetypal tug of war.

Story as Medicine for Couples

Jungian analyst and storyteller Clarissa Pinkola-Estes says stories are medicine that contain their own remedies. They help patients reclaim what they have lost or forgotten or repair what is broken. Stories "do not require that we do, be, act, anything—we need only listen."[35] Her emphasis on story follows Jung, who says that many patients come to analysis because they have a story no one knows of and that has never been told, not even to their most intimate friends—or their partner. Jung believes that "therapy only really begins after the investigation of that wholly personal story."[36] The story alone illustrates the partner's background; it is "the crucial thing."[37]

Telling one's story to an empathic listener reverberates through the entire bodymind. For instance, patients may take their first deep, long exhale as an agonizing silence is broken. Sometimes, rigidity dissolves into tears at the end of a telling. Breaking open and dissolving are apt images for the visible transformation of protective armor.[38] Defenses against the terror of speaking dissolve, at least for a time. Such moments often indicate a genuine break-*through* in response to break*down*, and are often turning points in therapy. When a partner softens—physically, emotionally, mentally, and spiritually—they become open to other ways of seeing and being together.

Therapists shed different light on entrenched archetypal patterns by helping couples reimagine their story. They can interrupt a story to re-enliven it by asking questions: *Wait. Slow down. Go back. How old were you when this happened? What else do you remember about that moment? Looking back on it now, what would you say to your younger self?* Addressing the other partner: *How much of this story did you know? Hearing it now, what comes to mind? What's going on inside of you?* To both partners: *What new thoughts, feelings, or sensations are coming to mind for both of you?* Telling the story anew, or re-storying, introduces meaningful new images, insights, and emotions. Everyone participating creatively in the moment experiences the soul's natural aliveness, its inclination towards movement. "Nowhere is the movement or the sense of life of the psyche seen more clearly than in story, which moves images and affects towards a satisfying end that resonates within us."[39] As the story changes to reflect deeper and fuller truths, so do the partners and their relationship.

The act of telling one's story also introduces another archetypal pair with deep roots in the human psyche, Narrator/Audience. In individual therapy, the dynamic relationship between narrator and audience is embodied in at least three ways. First, the patient tells their story aloud, listening to themselves. Next, the patient speaks to the therapist, the most immediate external audience. Finally, the patient is also speaking to the soul, for the soul, too, is listening. "The power of story and metaphor (like art, dance or music)" says Corbett, can "move the soul much more directly than the same ideas expressed as an abstract concept or interpretation."[40]

In couples therapy, there is another crucially important audience for the story: one's partner. Evoking the deepest layers of a personal story is slow, patient work, sometimes made more difficult by the presence of an intimate partner. Telling a story that has never been told to them may be the most fearful part of the endeavor since it is a moment of acute vulnerability. When working with couples, rather than pressing for stories to be told, it is important to trust the wisdom of the person holding the story because some partners may be unwilling or unable to hear them. Others are not ready to hear them, and some cannot be trusted with them because they weaponize these stories for use in later conflicts. Aware of the archetypal power of story, therapists also respect the wisdom of the story itself, knowing that it can only be told when *it* is ready. They will wait patiently and wonder with the couple, *What stories are here that are not yet ready to be told?*

Chickasaw poet Linda Hogan says, "story is a power that describes our world, our human being, sets out the rules and intricate laws of human beings in relationship with all the rest."[41] The act of telling the wholly personal story can mean admitting to oneself and to one's partner the often unspoken and unacknowledged assumptions and fantasies of relationship. For example, *When I'm sick I want you to wrap me in a blanket and bring a cup of hot cocoa like my dad did.* Or, *I wish you would give me space when I'm angry or upset and trust me to work it out alone.*

Therapists witness the ways in which couples endlessly revise their stories to reflect deeper understanding. Like a novel in process, events get edited, embellished, and rearranged. Partners speak from a particular and limited point of view, not the omniscient view. Since none of us is God, we all are partial narrators able to tell only part of the story. Yet, as L. L. Whyte said, "one of the dangers of our age, more damaging than ever before, is *total obsession with partial ideas.*"[42] Therapists confront this danger whenever one of the partners insists that their story of an event is the whole truth and nothing but. Literalism is a prison that confines therapeutic work, effectively bringing it to a standstill. It is a movement against soul and the soul's natural inclination to move. The task is not to fix the story, but instead "to expand and deepen the story, thus releasing the energy bound within it."[43]

Partners caught in conflict and stuck in their own story are often embodying just one pole of an archetype. Each person believes their version of a story and cannot see it differently. In such situations, therapists feel pressured to assume the role of judge. A more generative approach is to assume that *both* narratives are correct; both partners are telling the truth, *their* truth. As partners retell their versions again, therapists can slow the narratives and ask nuanced, detailed questions. *What was it like to tell the story this time? Are there things you didn't say this time that you want to share now?* It can be very difficult for the other partner to sit and listen without interrupting, verbally or nonverbally, and refrain from interjecting. Inviting the partner's awareness, therapists can ask: *How was it for you to sit and listen to this? What did you hear your partner say? Even if you don't agree with it—at all—can you see how your partner may have felt or why they reacted this way?* This work helps to remind couples of just how differently each partner takes in and experiences things, and it reinforces each other's uniqueness and complexity.

The archetypal spirit in story and storytelling is embodied in Clio, one of the nine muses in the Greek tradition. As the goddess of history, Clio presents tales of the soul as if they were facts. "We are caught in our stories, the soul's histories, tragedies, comedies, its need to form its subjectivity as history."[44] When couples tell their stories, it dignifies the events. It also represents attempts to make sense of things that are painful, confusing, or overwhelming by creating order out of chaos. Stories may also be slender footholds of stability for partners and couples. Narratives hold us (together), so it is hard sometimes to release them for fear of the unknown. However, it is possible to strengthen (tighten) the foothold and, paradoxically, expand (loosen) it at the same time by anchoring narratives in their archetypal foundations. The meaningfulness of events becomes personal and more-than-personal when couples can shift a literal event "halfway back toward the once-upon-a-time, toward the sacred and eternal."[45]

Excursion: Becoming a Vulnerable Observer

Couples come to therapy hoping for progress, which places pressure on therapists to create progress. A Jungian approach questions the word *progress* itself. Progress towards what? Progress for the ego looks very different to progress for the soul—if *soul* and *progress* even belong in the same sentence—because couples and therapists engage with inner figures whose autonomous needs "may radically alter, even dominate, our thoughts and feelings."[46] When everyone treats the figures crowding the room as persons, not objects, couples therapy becomes risky, playful, and spontaneous. "One doesn't know what they're up to or what they'll do or say next."[47] The improvisational quality of the work, in which nothing goes to plan, is "the soul's answer to egocentricity."[48]

Therapists comfortable with improvisation may detect nuances within repetitive patterns or an opening in the couple's story where fresh understandings can emerge. They might invite the partner-narrator to begin *Once upon a time...* or to imagine themselves as singers who "receive the other as if he were music, listening to the rhythm and cadence of his tale, its thematic repetitions, and the disharmonies."[49] Then everyone in the clinical space can "become mythologists of the psyche, that is, students of the tales of the soul, as mythology originally means 'storytelling.' If the soul is a chord only the ear can reveal it."[50]

Repair, insight, and understanding may emerge from the work. Growth is possible for couples, too, so long as therapists remember that growth is not strictly an additive process, and neither does it fit a timetable. Anne Ulanov suggests a different idea of growth: Therapist and partners circumambulate an idea, an image, an intuition or a felt sense, conceiving it together. Such a process "usually takes place in stillness and darkness ... the world of the unseen, and the mysterious processes of the unconscious where creative activity starts."[51] The ability to enter the darkness with the couple means surrendering many of the labels, props, and goals that structure therapeutic work. In doing so, therapists become what anthropologist Ruth Behar referred to as a vulnerable observer, allowing the couple sitting in front of you to break your heart.[52]

Couples and the Underworld

As implied throughout this book, a Jungian approach to couples therapy extends beyond cognitive-behavioral psychologies that aim for social adaptation. Jung's archetypal approach seeks wisdom in the unconscious, which is often portrayed in myth as an underworld. Therapists accompany the suffering couple into the dark and disorienting underworld depths, the realm of the dead, and of death, and of transformation. The descent to the underworld, an archetypal motif found in many cultures around the world, dramatizes the soul's special relationship with death—a relationship that bestows significance and meaning on the couple's suffering.[53]

"To study soul, we must go deep, and when we go deep, soul becomes involved," says Hillman, because "the logos of the soul, psychology, implies the act of travelling the soul's labyrinth in which we can never go deep enough."[54] The Romantic poet John Keats describes the world as "the vale of soul-making."[55] *Vale* is an antique word for a valley, often imagined in world mythologies as the underworld. They are places of great quiet, where one can slow down, feel the presence of the Self, and listen to the soul speaking. Soul-making, implies Keats, happens *in* the world not beyond it, wherever we are profoundly, bodily, and emotionally committed. Relationships, too, are just such places.

"The underworld realm of the dead ... is also the fecund ground from which new life emerges, a place of healing, initiation, and revelation."[56] Mythologist Lans Smith elaborates this idea while focusing on stories of descent as marriage narratives. Inanna's descent to the Great Below (Sumerian), Isis and Osiris (Egyptian), the Homeric Hymn to Demeter (Greek). and Eros and Psyche (Roman) "transmit a millennial wisdom about life and marriage which we should not ignore."[57] The underworld for the ancients "was a dual realm, part hell, and part heaven," Smith says, "like marriage. Like any relationship that lasts longer than three months."[58] Descent narratives affirm that the deepest, most soulful relationships are formed and re-formed through surprising events that draw us down, out of busy social life. The shocking nature of the descent calls to mind Jung's statement about encounters with the Self as a defeat for the ego discussed in Chapter 1. The sting of defeat may be especially sharp and necessary for someone with a controlling ego who seemingly directs their life (and their partner's life) with the illusion that they have a firm grip on the reins. For them, it is a symbolic death, an underworld experience, and it is often profoundly disorienting.

In a sense, couples therapists are death doulas, trained in the emotional, spiritual, and psychological dimensions of endings—sometimes of relationships, but more commonly, of ways of thinking, behaving, or being. Mythic stories of descent to the underworld, the archetypal journey toward symbolic death, may be especially relevant to couples living between old and new ways of being together. Perhaps all first marriages, the first idealized fantasies of life together, must die to make way for a second and more real union—with the same partner, in many cases. "The soul favours the death experience to usher in change."[59] What else motivates couples to enter therapy than the sense that something profound has changed—or needs to? Yet death is not anti-life; instead, "it may be a demand for an encounter with absolute reality, a demand for a fuller life through the death experience" because "until we can choose death, we cannot choose life."[60]

Conclusion

Working in the depths with couples, therapists develop an archetypal sensibility: A way of being, thinking, listening, and imagining in mythic patterns, the deep and ancient foundation of collective human experience. Hillman describes psychology as mythology in modern dress.[61] He emphasizes its archetypal dimension to help people deepen into their experiences and find meaning in their recurring patterns. Archetypally, our lives and our relationships are mythic. Joseph Campbell reminds us, "the continued romance of Beauty and the Beast stands this afternoon on the corner of Forty-second Street and Fifth Avenue, waiting for the light to change."[62]

Archetypal energies are responsible for the ties that bind couples together, and they are also the forces that tear them apart. Yet few therapists begin their careers thinking archetypally and in mythic terms. Rather, they are often dragged to it, seeking relief from the depths of a couple's misery and needing new, more spacious ways to imagine relational dynamics. Edward Edinger, in his aptly titled book *The Eternal Drama*, describes mythology as "the self-revelation of the archetypal psyche" that provides "the objective foundation for personal psychology."[63] For artists, poets, and psychotherapists, mythology is "a treasury of images used in their craft."[64] Therapists who recognize the dramatic motifs in couples' stories and feel their mythic resonance can skillfully address these powerful archetypal energies. Rooting them in the foundations of the psyche creates a bridge to ancient ways of knowing and being, a reminder of the presence of soul in therapeutic work and in the life of individuals, couples, communities, cultures, and the world.

Notes

1 Jung 1959.
2 Hillman 1979, p. 200.
3 Hillman 1979, p. 200.
4 Hillman 1979, p. 200.
5 Jung 1959.
6 Jung1954, para. 155.
7 Jung 1954, para. 155.
8 Jung 1953, para. 109.
9 Jung 1936, para. 395.
10 Jung 1953, para. 109.

11 Jung 1919, para. 280.
12 Jung 1953, para. 109.
13 Hillman 2013, p. 23.
14 Hillman 2013, p. 23.
15 Hillman 1997, p. 83.
16 Hillman 1997, p. 72.
17 Archetypes are bipolar in another, more fundamental way. Jung uses the metaphor of the light spectrum to describe the archetype's two poles: the red somatic/instinctual end and the blue mental/psychic end. In his late work he developed the concept of the *psychoid* to link body (instinct) and psyche (image), saying it is "fairly probable ... that psyche and matter are two different aspects of one and the same thing" (Jung 1946, para. 418). Fundamentally, "instincts and images have the same psychoid root" (Samuels, Shorter, & Plaut 1986, p. 30).
18 Jung 1963, para. 706.
19 Jung 1963, para. 706.
20 Jung 1963, para. 706.
21 Hillman 1978, p. 159.
22 Sells 2000, p. 20.
23 See Watkins 1986 and Casey 1974.
24 Jung 1971, para. 84.
25 For further reading, see *Invisible Guests* by Mary Watkins (1986) or Edward Casey's 1974 essay "Toward an archetypal imagination."
26 Readers already familiar with Hillman's work will recognize that we are referring to *psychologizing*, one of the four natural moves of the psyche he describes in *Re-Visioning Psychology*. Psychologizing is "seeing through" any idea, event, story, or action taken as the only, exclusive *literal* truth to its deeper, symbolic meanings.
27 Jung 1964.
28 Jung 1964, para. 523.
29 Campbell 2008[1949].
30 Jung 1931, para 789.
31 Jung 1977, p. 348.
32 As just two examples, see Smith 2003 and Wolkstein 1991.
33 Jung 1916, para. 18.
34 Hillman 1977, p. 65.
35 Pinkola-Estes 1992, p. 15.
36 Jung 1989[1961], p. 117.
37 Jung 1989[1961], p. 124.
38 Reich 1973[1945].
39 Corbett 1996, p. 85.
40 Corbett 1996, p. 92.
41 Hogan 1998, p. 9.
42 Whyte 1978, p. 8; original italics.
43 Houston 1997, p. 99.
44 Hillman 1983, p. 43.
45 Hillman 1983, p. 45.
46 Hillman 1983, p. 55.
47 Coppin & Nelson 2017, p. 186.
48 Hillman 1975, p. 32.
49 Hillman 1994, pp. 22–23.
50 Hillman 1994, pp. 22–23.
51 Ulanov 1971, pp. 170–171.
52 Behar 1996.

53 Hillman 1975, p. xiv.
54 Hillman 1979, p. 25.
55 Keats 1992, p. 249.
56 ARAS 2018, n. p.
57 Smith 2003, p. 7.
58 Smith 2003, p. 7.
59 Hillman 1997, p. 68.
60 Hillman 1997, pp. 62–63.
61 Hillman 1979, pp. 23–24.
62 Campbell 2008[1949], p. 2.
63 Edinger 2001, p. 2.
64 Edinger 2001, p. 2.

References

ARAS. (September 2018). Serpent. *Archive for research in archetypal symbolism* [newsletter] www.aras.org.
Behar, R. (1996). *The vulnerable observer*. University of Michigan.
Campbell, J. (2008). *The hero with a thousand faces* (3rd ed.). New World Library. (Original work published 1949.)
Casey, E. (1974). Toward an archetypal imagination. *Spring*, 1–32.
Coppin, J. & Nelson, E. (2017). *The art of inquiry* (3rd exp. ed.). Spring Publications.
Corbett, L. (1996). *The religious function of the psyche*. Routledge.
Edinger, E. (2001). *The eternal drama: The inner meaning of Greek mythology*. Shambhala.
Hillman, J. (1975). *Re-visioning psychology*, rev. ed. HarperPerennial.
Hillman, J. (1977). An inquiry into image. *Spring*, 62–88.
Hillman, J. (1978). Further notes on image. *Spring*, 152–182.
Hillman, J. (1979). *The dream and the underworld*. Harper & Row.
Hillman, J.(1983) *Healing fiction*. Spring Publications.
Hillman, J. (1994). *Insearch: Psychology and Religion*. Spring Publications.
Hillman, J. (1997). *Suicide and the soul* (2nd ed.). Spring Publications.
Hillman, J. (2013). *Archetypal psychology: Uniform edition of the works of James Hillman* (Vol. 1). Spring Publications.
Hogan, L. (1998). First people. In L. Hogan, D. Metzger, & B. Peterson (Eds.), *Intimate nature* (pp. 6–19). Fawcett Books.
Houston, J. (1997). *The search for the beloved* (2nd ed.). Jeremy Tarcher.
Jung, C. G. (1916). Two kinds of thinking. *CW* 5.
Jung, C. G. (1919). Instinct and unconscious. *CW* 8.
Jung, C. G. (1931). The stages of life. *CW* 8.
Jung, C. G. (1936). Wotan. *CW* 10.
Jung, C. G. (1946). On the nature of the psyche. *CW* 10.
Jung, C. G. (1953). Two essays on analytical psychology. *CW* 7.
Jung, C. G. (1954). Psychological aspects of the mother archetype. *CW* 9i.
Jung, C. G. (1959). The archetypes and the collective unconscious. *CW* 9i.
Jung, C. G. (1963). Mysterium coniunctionis. *CW* 14.
Jung, C. G. (1964). The symbolic life. *CW* 18.
Jung, C. G. (1971). Psychological types. *CW* 6.

Jung, C. G. (1977). *C. G. Jung speaking* (W. McGuire & R. F. C. Hull, Eds.). Princeton University Press.

Jung, C. G. (1989). *Memories, dreams, reflections* (A. Jaffé, Ed.; R. Winston & C. Winston, Trans.; Rev. ed.). Vintage. (Original work published 1961.)

Keats, J. (1992). *Letters of John Keats*. Oxford University Press.

Pinkola-Estes, C. (1992). *Women who run with the wolves*. Ballantine.

Reich, W. (1973). *Character analysis* (V. Carfagno, Trans.; 3rd ed.). WRM Press. (Original work published 1945.)

Samuels, A., Shorter, B., & Plaut, F. (Eds.). (1986). *A critical dictionary of Jungian analysis*. Routledge.

Sells, B. (Ed.). (2000). *Working with images*. Spring Publications.

Smith, E. L. (2003). *Sacred mysteries*. Blue Dolphin Publishing.

Ulanov, A. (1971). *The feminine in Jungian psychology and in Christian theology*. Northwestern University Press.

Watkins, M. (1986). *Invisible guests*. The Analytic Press.

Whyte, L. L. (1978). *The unconscious before Freud*. St. Martin's Press.

Wolkstein, D. (1991). *The first love stories*. HarperCollins.

Chapter 4

Typology in Couples Therapy

Many therapists are familiar with moments when couples in therapy realize, perhaps for the first time, they are not alike—at all. And with this realization comes anger, frustration, and heartbreak. Their binding spell of enchantment has been broken, and complaints burst forth quickly for both of them: *The things I used to love about you are driving me crazy now ... I used to love your sense of humor, but now you are just another child that I have to deal with ... You used to be my rock, but now you don't have a feeling bone in your body ... We couldn't keep our hands off each other but now we live like roommates ... We fight over the stupidest things ... Everything is irritating ... When I am driving, you always chime in because you think your way is best ... You know I like to be on time, yet you are always causing us to be late ... I am sick of you overscheduling us all the time. I need some quiet time ... Who loads a dishwasher like that? ...*

These types of exchanges between couples are examples of Jung's typology on full display. Such relational dynamics surface in nearly all committed relationships that last beyond the initial honeymoon period. Jung's typology highlights and accounts for these profound shifts in the felt sense of one another as couples are dragged from the heights of love down into the pits of misery. Familiarity with the basics of Jung's typology is useful for helping couples understand what is going on between them at this stage of their relationship and what they can do about it.

In 1921, Jung published *Psychological Types*, calling it "the fruit of nearly twenty years' work in the domain of practical psychology."[1] In this groundbreaking text, Jung introduces the basic attitudes of *introversion* and *extraversion* and distinguishes the four mental functions, *sensing, thinking, feeling, and intuiting*, seating them in a meta-framework to make sense of the wide variations in how people experience themselves, each other, and the world. Typology, he argues, "determines and limits a person's judgment" from the very outset of life.[2] Over a century later, this work continues to be published and translated into numerous languages; its psychological perspective still resonant the world over. Despite such widespread acceptance, Jung's typological theory and its practical applications are often overlooked by therapists today, even those with Jungian training.

DOI: 10.4324/9781032688008-5

Perhaps typology slips so easily from conscious awareness because it is foundational in the personality. We may function along in our typologies as unaware as fish are of water. Jung introduced so many other shimmering ideas and concepts (alchemy, archetypes, the collective unconscious, synchronicity, the transcendent function) that typology, that ubiquitous matrix, fades from the foreground. And yet in couples therapy, fuller awareness and appreciation for innate typologies, typological limitations, and typological differences relieve relational pressure.

Psychological Types also spawned an entire personality testing industry,[3] beginning with the Gray-Wheelwright Jungian Type Survey designed in the 1930s (now updated as the Gray-Wheelwright-Winer Test), the Singer-Loomis Type Deployment Inventory, the Keirsey Temperament Sorter, and the Myers-Briggs Type Indicator,[4] which, having been taken by over 50 million people, is the most widely used personality test in history.[5] Jung's theory of typology is so accepted in the mainstream that even those who haven't had any personality testing have some understanding of where they are on the introversion–extraversion continuum and can make some distinction between themselves and their partners as to degrees of thinking and feeling.

This chapter provides a basic introduction to Jung's typology theory and its use in couples therapy. It cannot address the subtleties and complexity of Jung's 600-page text. Nor can proper attention be given to the expert amplifications by John Beebe,[6] Daryl Sharp,[7] Angelo Spoto,[8] Marie-Louise von Franz and James Hillman,[9] and Joseph Wheelwright,[10] to name just a few. As with any general introduction, this chapter makes necessary oversimplifications and omissions while inviting the reader to explore typology at more nuanced levels using the primary sources.

Two Basic Attitudes: Extraversion and Introversion

Jung lays the foundation for his psychology of types by introducing the term *attitude* as "a readiness of the psyche to act or react in a certain way."[11] Attitudes include anything and everything influencing the psyche, including "innate disposition, environmental influences, experiences in life, insights, and convictions gained through differentiation, collective views, etc."[12] With this, Jung delineates two basic typological attitudes, extraversion and introversion, as poles on a continuum describing how one relates to their inner and outer worlds.

Extraversion is "a mode of psychological orientation where the movement of energy is toward the outer world."[13] Extraverts are energized by being engaged out in the world and with others. They can enjoy doing many different things at once. They like to influence others and their environment, and they want to be influenced by them as well.[14] Spending time alone can be draining for extraverts. While extraverts value their outer connections, they can also fear their inner world because they generally have less access to it.[15] Extraverts, being so at ease in an extraverted world, can also have some fear of introverts, finding them withdrawn, intense, or weird.[16]

At the other end of the continuum, the introverted attitude is "a mode of psychological orientation where the movement of energy is toward the inner world."[17] Introverts enjoy solitude and recharge by being alone. Because the inner world is the real world for introverts, they tend to be more in touch with internal resources and better understand themselves.[18] Introverts tend to feel like outsiders in an extraverted world. They may find extraverts intrusive or exhausting. At extremes, Wheelwright noted that they can be egotistic and domineering, trying to impose their inner world onto those around them. Because anything outside of themselves feels foreign, introverts may have some fear of others and also struggle with their agency in the world.

It is difficult for strong introverts and extraverts to conceive of just how differently they experience themselves and the world. Review Table 4.1 and see where you and your loved ones most naturally fit on this continuum.

Normalizing each person's basic attitude, introversion or extraversion, and noting a couple's differences can often ease tension when working with frustrated partners. It is helpful for couples to use the language of introversion and extraversion to effectively communicate preferences for staying in, going out, being alone, or sharing time together. Helping couples voice typological differences inherently reframes feelings of rejection, selfishness, overwhelm, or abandonment. For example, a strongly extraverted partner may schedule many weekend activities, while an introverted partner may prefer quiet time at home. Having them identify their needs and preferences according to their basic attitudes allows each partner to be seen, heard, and understood. The extravert is honored and can enjoy the fullness of activity, while the introvert has permission for solitude with the freedom to join in as desired. Have couples review Table 4.1 and see how they identify themselves and each other.

Table 4.1 The Basic Attitudes of Introversion and Extraversion

More introverted if you ...	*More extraverted if you ...*
Have a rich inner life. View life from the inside out.	Are primarily interested in and concerned with the external world.
Gain energy through inner reflection and solitude.	Gain energy from socializing and being out and about.
Get more excited by ideas than by external activities.	Find your energy is depleted when spending too much time alone.
Prefer a few deep, close relationships to many casual ones.	Feel confident, friendly, and assertive, having many friends and acquaintances.
Feel tired and drained after socializing, even if it is enjoyable.	Prefer talking with someone rather than sitting alone and thinking.
Listen well and expect others to do the same.	Are always on the go.
Think first and talk later.	Think *as* you speak.
Express yourself well in writing.	Express yourself well verbally.

Four Mental Functions

Jung divides all mental functioning into four categories: sensing, thinking, feeling, and intuiting.[19] The sensing function *"registers reality as real"* and provides a sensation of what *is*.[20] Next, the thinking function classifies or defines what is being sensed or perceived. The feeling function then judges or *"assigns a value* to the thing that has been perceived and named."[21] Finally, the intuiting function provides *"implications or possibilities* for what has been empirically perceived, logically defined and discriminatingly evaluated."[22] Jung classifies the thinking and feeling as rational *judging* functions because they use logical, reflective, linear processes to arrive at conclusions. Whereas sensing and intuiting are nonrational *perceiving* functions providing immediate, non-linear means to arrive at conclusions to determine what is, what was, or what may be. When using the sensing or intuiting function, "the physical perception of something does not depend on logic—things just *are*."[23] Thus, these functions are not "something *contrary* to reason, but something *beyond* reason."[24]

The sensation function "mediates the perception of a physical stimulus."[25] Whether filtered through an introverted or extraverted attitude, it provides a measure of reality as it is *right now*.[26] Strong sensing types can be "factual and very observant, and they are capable of not only 'seeing' but of remembering those facts and details."[27] They seem to have an extra measure of common sense and are often considered practical and down to earth.

The thinking function follows its own laws, bringing together "the contents of ideation into conceptual connection with one another."[28] Thinking can be active or passive, directed or free-floating. The result of any kind of thinking is a logical conclusion or judgment. "Thinking-types tend to be impersonal or firm minded, and can be argumentative, critical, or blunt in their human relationships."[29] When speaking with a strong thinker, one can come away with a feeling of being criticized or corrected, even when that is not the thinker's intention. When one partner in a relationship is a strong thinker, therapists can assist in teasing out this felt sense in how they communicate, making it more conscious. The thinker will become more aware of *how* their communications are being received, and their partner can be mindful of being in the presence of a strong thinking function.

The feeling function uses subjective evaluation to arrive at conclusions.[30] Strong feelers get their answers instantly, unlike thinkers who must do mental calculus to arrive at answers. However, emotions can often cloud the feeling function. Additionally, in relationships, strong thinkers may discount the value of their partner's feelings as *just being emotional*. However, "when it is differentiated it [the feeling function] is not emotional at all."[31] If a couple is awash in affect, a typologically attuned therapist can help strong feelers sort out what they are truly feeling from their emotions.

The intuiting function "mediates perceptions in an *unconscious way*."[32] With intuition, viable solutions and ideas arrive whole and complete. For example, a thinker constructs a building from the ground up. (*Logically*, a thinker would agree, *for how else does one build a building other than brick by brick?*) But something very different happens for an intuitive: a perfectly completed building simply arrives in the mind. (*Of course*, the intuitive would agree, *for how else can one build a building unless one can see it first?*)

Typological differences are most easily recognized in couples' bickering over how to do home projects, organize the refrigerator, or when planning a trip. At first blush, these never-ending differences of opinion appear petty and nitpicking, but they are the unacknowledged typological differences eroding intimacy and connection. Helping couples recognize their typological differences can help dissolve long-held battles over correctness or competence and invite respect and wonder.

The natural development (or overdevelopment) of some functions comes at the expense of the development of others. Jung does not privilege one function over another, though cultures often do. They are simply different ways of taking in and making sense of the world, each with distinct advantages and disadvantages. However, Jung does place sensing, thinking, feeling, and intuiting into a hierarchy relative to the degree of conscious access an individual has to each function (see Figure 4.1).

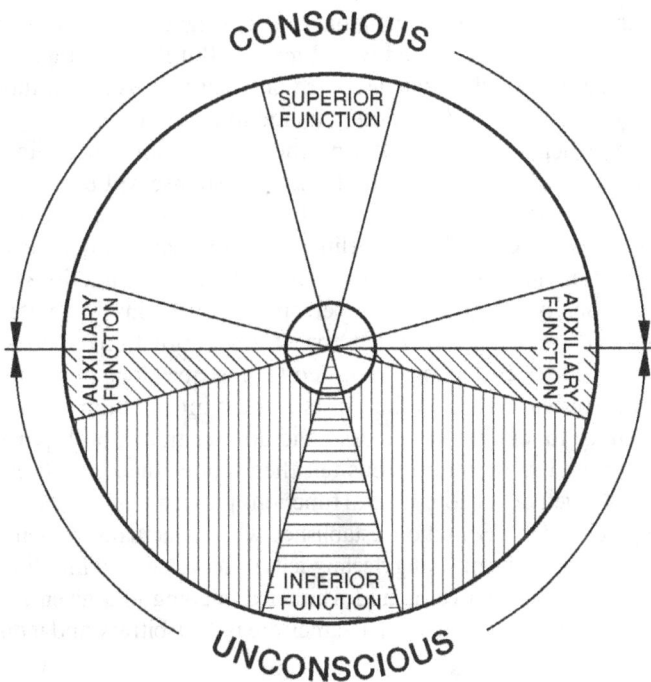

Figure 4.1 Hierarchy of Functions. Adapted from *Analytical Psychology* (p. 128), by C. G. Jung, 1989. Princeton University Press. Copyright 1989 by Princeton University Press. Adapted with permission.

Someone's superior function is usually readily available and most consciously accessible. Conversely, the inferior function is the least consciously available. These functions can be likened to satellite dishes picking up and processing information. The superior function would be the largest and most powerful dish, while the inferior function would be smallest and weakest. The auxiliary functions vary in size, somewhere between the superior and inferior. For example, a person with a superior thinking function often has little access to their inferior feeling function. However, they do have some conscious access to their auxiliary sensation and intuition functions.

To discover a couple's superior and inferior functions, typologically attuned therapists are more intentional with their choice of verbs when asking couples questions and pay close attention to the verbs used by partners as they respond. For example, asking a strong thinker with an inferior feeling function what they *think* about a situation they usually reply with a litany of *I think* ... responses and provide logical, coherent, and detailed answers. (Often, much to their own satisfaction.) However, when probing further and asking that same thinker what they *feel* about some aspect of the situation they just described, they typically respond in one of two ways. Sometimes, they will appear to be perplexed by the question and have trouble finding words for a response. In other cases, a question about how they feel elicits further *I think* ... , similar in nature to their original response. Sometimes, a superior thinker may even respond with *I feel* .... But if the therapist pays close attention to what is said, they will discover that what follows are all thoughts, *not* feelings, albeit with a little more emotion to add to the confusion.

Conversely, when therapists ask a partner with a superior feeling function what they actually *think* about a situation, the response will usually be a series of *I feel* ... statements. Again, if the therapist pays close attention to the material response, they will find feelings, not thoughts. Since partners in a relationship often have differing superior and inferior functions, therapists should intentionally expand their repertoire of questions to invite information, if available, from all four functions. If a superior thinker does not have conscious access to their feelings, repeated feeling questions only frustrate and alienate them. Instead, attuned therapists can get information from the much-needed auxiliary functions. In this case, therapists can ask both partners what their *intuitions* and *sense* impressions tell them about their situation.

When taken together, the four mental functions provide a comprehensive view of reality. Jung reiterates, "Sensation establishes what is actually present, thinking enables us to recognize its meaning, feeling tells us its value, and intuition points to possibilities as to whence it came and whither it is going in a given situation."[33] Likened to the four points on a compass, they are both arbitrary and indispensable.

Eight Psychological Types

Jung also noticed that the two basic attitudes of extraversion and introversion influence how each mental function operates.[34] Therefore, he further divides each mental function into two types. For example, there are two kinds of thinking: extraverted thinking and introverted thinking. With this, Jung arrives at his formulation of eight psychological types:

Sensing (perceiving)	Extraverted Sensing (1)
	Introverted Sensing (2)
Thinking (judging)	Extraverted Thinking (3)
	Introverted Thinking (4)
Feeling (judging)	Extraverted Feeling (5)
	Introverted Feeling (6)
Intuiting (perceiving)	Extraverted Intuiting (7)
	Introverted Intuiting (8)

An individual has varying degrees of conscious access to these eight psychological types. While reading the following descriptions of each one, notice which are most familiar and which seem most foreign. These will be clues to your superior and inferior functions. While reading, pay attention to any loved ones, friends, colleagues, or couples who come to mind. Share this section with someone who knows you best and take some educated guesses about each other's superior and inferior functions. Notice the rich conversation that follows. However, resist the temptation to simplify yourself or others with reductive all-or-nothing thinking. Find hints and shades of yourself in as many types as possible. These will be your auxiliary functions.

To help highlight the differences between the eight psychological types, the discussion below characterizes them as if they were operating in the psyche as the superior function.

Extraverted and Introverted Sensing

For the extraverted sensing type, reality is external and concrete. They sense things directly and often have a very accurate understanding of things as they exist. They have a robust and sensual tie to the outside world.[35] Extraverted sensers are often committed to living life to the fullest. They are punctual, adept people who read maps easily, rarely lose things or get lost, or forget appointments. They are great at parties and love beautiful things and beautiful people. At the extreme, strong extraverted sensers can get lost in the now, becoming exploitative and overly hedonistic.[36]

An introverted sensing type, on the other hand, bases perceptions on their unique, subjective experience. They stand apart and allow their experience of the other to percolate through their own subjectivity.[37] Others can confuse their quiet and calm presence for connection, but they are often unavailable and attuned internally.[38] Jung adds that because of this inner orientation, strong introverted sensers, while looking and playing their part, often leave their partners (and therapists) confused and with a sense of feeling devalued.

Review the lists in Table 4.2 to determine if your sensing function is more consciously extraverted or introverted.

Have couples review the lists in Table 4.2 and facilitate a conversation. Help them notice the similarities and differences in how they sense things.

Extraverted and Introverted Thinking

An extraverted thinking type orders life "in accordance with logical conclusions arrived at through consideration of facts or ideas grounded in objective experience and generally accepted principles."[39] Extraverted thinkers accumulate and value facts. Their psychological processes are directed and intellectual, using thoughts as tools to serve their purpose.[40] They are concerned with generally accepted broader truths. A person overly dominated by extraverted thinking can become overbearing, inflexible, or intolerant. With little

Table 4.2 Extraverted and Introverted Sensing

Extraverted Sensing	Introverted Sensing
Externally oriented perceiving process focused on the present.	An internal process of perceiving.
Uses the senses (seeing, hearing, smelling, touching, tasting) to get external information.	Gets information about internal physical sensations, images, or dialogue without evaluation or logical analysis.
Rarely fights facts. Accepts what is perceived in whatever form it takes.	Has an enduring perspective that shapes their view of the world and their relationships.
A deep-seated sense of the reality of the external world. Realistic. Rarely makes factual errors.	Experiences their inner reality as amazingly real and adheres to it even when at odds with others.
Assimilates details. Provides comprehensive descriptions of what has been perceived.	Sustains highly articulated internal images, often with timeless characteristics.
Excels at activities demanding attention to detail.	Strongly trusts their gut reaction.
Unusually open-minded. Relatively unprejudiced, patient, and egalitarian.	Detailed descriptions of internal images or physical experiences often provide new awareness or insight.
Aesthetic taste. Savors the present moment. Enjoys the good things in life (food, art, music, sports, sex, nature).	Robust aesthetic appreciation, often for abstract forms of art.
Love is based on physical attraction.	Vivid memory. Exceptional recall. Uses past experience as a guide to making present decisions.

access to their unconscious feeling function, they may lack sympathy for others, making it difficult in partnerships or family situations. They may also have little understanding, tolerance, or respect for those with more access to the other ways of knowing.[41]

The introverted thinking type is also strongly influenced by ideas, but those ideas are grounded in their own subjective foundations rather than external, objective data.[42] Their linear process-oriented thinking relies on internal, subjective logic to arrive at conclusions. Introverted thinkers value the ideas that arise from their internal processing more than external logic.[43] Introverted thinkers are concerned with the logic and conviction of their own inner truths.[44] Their introverted thinking can cause them to appear stubborn or hardheaded to their partner, and their unique conclusions may lead to misunderstandings. Strong introverted thinkers also tend to believe they are the smartest people in the room or that everyone else is stupid.[45]

Review the lists in Table 4.3 and determine if your thinking tends to be more consciously extraverted or introverted.

Have couples review the lists in Table 4.3 and facilitate a conversation. Help them notice the similarities and differences in how they think.

When working with couples, strong extraverted thinkers can be identified in the countertransference when one begins to feel lectured to by a

Table 4.3 Extraverted and Introverted Thinking

Extraverted Thinking	*Introverted Thinking*
Uses impersonal logic to weigh pros and cons and draw conclusions.	Takes a logical but unconventional approach to complicated tasks.
Applies causal logic to everything and everyone. *If…(this), then…(conclusion).*	Gets satisfaction from thinking seriously about something and reaching a conclusion.
Precise use of words to provide detailed accounts of events and circumstances.	Creates unique words and labels or changes ideas to satisfy personal considerations.
Seeks unbiased meaning in their own life and the world around them.	The internal world is usually alive with abstract ideas.
Perfectionistic. Orderliness and stability are preferred. Planning is essential for all things. Seldom acts spontaneously.	Likes working independently. Relentless in carrying an idea or task to its conclusion. Practical applications are not important.
Governed by logic, not by emotions.	Finds new similarities between ideas, which lead to creative new ideas and conclusions.
Organizes to achieve practical, tangible goals. Seeks efficiency.	Is dedicated to reaching a thorough understanding of how things work.
Simplifies for clarity's sake.	Seeks to define the situation in a way that will be true in every eventuality.

teacher or when a partner complains of being made to feel like a child or finds themselves acting out. Strong introverted thinkers give detailed but sometimes faulty rationales for *how things should be.* Rather than inviting curiosity and dialogue, their partner (and even the therapist) can feel pressured into silent non-agreement or befuddlement and begin to experience themselves as dumb, naive, ineffectual, or powerless.

Extraverted and Introverted Feeling

The extraverted feeling type uses external objective data to measure and evaluate feeling.[46] Extraverted feelers like tradition, generally accepted values, and societal institutions. They enjoy collective expressions of culture, such as fashion trends, concerts, sporting events, and conventions.[47] Most extraverted feelers have an easy and genuine rapport with others. Because they are naturally attuned to the feelings and needs of others, extraverted feelers are quick to be self-sacrificing, making them good team players, co-workers, parents, and partners.

The introverted feeling type is a *still waters run deep* person who can be hard to read.[48] They feel all the time, and their feelings are often profound and intense. Introverted feelers can struggle to communicate these feelings. They can be silent, inaccessible, or hard to figure out.[49] They can lean toward melancholy and have little desire to impress or change others. At the extreme, some introverted feelers claim to know what others are thinking about them, usually imagining the worst.[50]

Review the lists in Table 4.4 to determine if your feeling function is more consciously extraverted or introverted.

Have couples review the lists in Table 4.4 and facilitate a conversation. Help them notice the similarities and differences in their feeling functions.

A superior extraverted feeler can be identified by their tendency to lose their own identity in relationships.[51] Therapists will notice this most overtly when one partner is overly attuned to the other at the expense of themselves. As a result, they often have great difficulty ending unhealthy relationships. Therapists can also help an introverted feeling partner notice how fast their mind jumps to conclusions about what the other may be thinking. Whether those conclusions are right or wrong, good communication for couples involves asking one another about their inner world, which includes information from as many functions as possible.

Extraverted and Introverted Intuiting

Jung describes the extraverted intuiting type as having "a keen nose for anything new and in the making."[52] Their "envisioning" process is always at work.[53] They can have a good sense of timing, knowing when to move forward and when to stop. They are often trend predictors with an

Table 4.4 Extraverted and Introverted Feeling

Extraverted Feeling	Introverted Feeling
Judging process keyed to the external world.	Uses unique internal standards to judge people and things.
Can be deeply concerned about social justice and events and circumstances at the boundaries between right and wrong.	Rational, one-step process of comparing situations with personal standards. Drawing conclusions is quick and straightforward.
Very emotionally warm, friendly, and sensitive to the wants and needs of others.	Often experiences themself as misunderstood.
Readily and consistently makes others feel valued and important.	Resists peer pressure or current trends. Can be overly idealistic when working for causes.
A remarkable number of friends and acquaintances. Diplomatic. Rarely tactless.	Very reliable and trustworthy. Stands by their word.
Quickly and skillfully engages people not seen for some time.	Can be reserved with affection and passion. Mysterious to others outside their circle.
Places high value on relationships.	May tend toward melancholy.
Does everything possible to avoid or minimize conflict.	When stressed, may become indifferent to others.

uncanny way of seeing what may emerge or recede in the culture. They make great talent scouts, developers, and travel planners. They can be inspiring visionaries.[54]

Introverted intuiting focuses primarily on inner psychic reality. Subjective impressions, imagery, and reverie dominate the mind of an introverted intuitive.[55] While using external objects as reference points, introverted intuitives do not concern themselves with external possibilities "but with what the external object has released within."[56] They have imaginations with few limitations, making them great poets, artists, prophets, and shamans.[57] Since the unconscious is the wellspring of these intuitive images and ideas, some introverted intuitives can have darker sides and ominous notions about the future. They may find it hard to communicate their inner visions and can often be misunderstood.

Review the lists in Table 4.5 to determine if your intuiting is more consciously extraverted or introverted.

Have couples review the lists in Table 4.5 and facilitate a conversation. Help them notice the similarities and differences in how their intuition functions.

Therapists will notice the presence of a strong introverted intuitive function when a partner remains firmly attached to their vision of the relationship despite overwhelming empirical evidence to the contrary. This can be seen when a

Table 4.5 Extraverted and Introverted Intuition

Extraverted Intuiting	*Introverted Intuiting*
Gets information about future possibilities but characteristically lacks detail.	Not time-bound, with many different insights into the past, present, or future, often leading to sweeping changes in understanding.
Not limited by logic or ethical evaluation.	Often, they use metaphors to explain their visions.
Visionaries leading themselves and others in new directions.	Insights about how external events may progress, including the future of relationships.
Perceives numerous new patterns that could arise from what is changing, stable, or ready to change.	A rich inner fantasy life with an almost unlimited imagination.
Thrives on complexity. Quick to propose a variety of imaginative solutions to issues or potential new uses for objects.	Experiences life from a variety of perspectives.
An unusual degree of spontaneity, innovation, and initiative. Non-conformist and versatile.	Welcomes change and embraces uncertainty. Nothing is final.
Little tolerance for situations that require detailed attention or careful follow-up. Looks to others for the next steps.	Generates new insights, many of which, however profound, are unfathomable or inconsequential.
Thrives on change. Easily adaptable.	Insights may be complicated and difficult to communicate to others.

couple has separated and is doing discernment therapy where one partner may be *so sure of reconciliation* even though the other partner moved out six months ago and is dating someone new. Because their inner visions are so powerful and seem so real, it can be difficult for strong introverted intuitives to realize that their vision is not *the* vision, but only one of many other possibilities.

The Inferior Function

The inferior function is the most unconscious, underdeveloped, and undifferentiated function. No introduction to typology is complete without discussing the inferior function's impact on individuals and relationships. It is particularly useful for therapists to have some working knowledge of the concept and its implications for themselves and their couples. On rare occasions when an individual does get to experience their inferior function, it can feel overwhelming, foreign, and even threatening.[58] "The essence of the inferior function is autonomy: it is independent, it attacks, it fascinates and so spins us about that we are no longer masters of ourselves and can no longer rightly distinguish between ourselves and others."[59] As an eruption from the unconscious, some even describe it as feeling like they are having an "inner breakdown."[60] Becoming overly sensitive can indicate the activation of the inferior function. In relationships, this can be the "psychological basis for discord and misunderstanding."[61]

For example, when a superior thinker with a feeling function in the inferior position experiences an eruption of feelings in therapy, the felt sense in the room is not one of *breakthrough* but of *breakdown*. And just as quickly, the superior thinker's feelings are gone. The trap door in the psyche from which these feelings suddenly emerged slams shut again, leaving everyone, including the superior thinker, in wonderment. Therapists and partners may mistakenly believe that the superior thinker now has regular access to that reservoir of feeling, but this is not the case. Once it shuts, that door, because it resides in the unconscious, cannot be located again until *it* decides to open again. This is most perplexing to partners who are strong feelers because of their continual and ready access to feelings. Since strong thinking partners get overwhelmed by these occasional eruptions of feelings, there is a tendency for partners to blame or pathologize them for their apparent *lack of willingness* to share their feelings when it is actually a matter of *lack of conscious access* to them.

Because the inferior function is so unconscious, it also catches our attention when we see it in others, creating attraction and intrigue, for it is truly undiscovered country. People are often attracted to others who possess in abundance those functions that are less developed in themselves. Typologically, introverts are often drawn to extraverts. Strong feelers enchant strong thinkers. The clichéd phrase, *You complete me*, is entirely accurate, typologically speaking. However, with one partner's inferior function leaning so heavily on the other's superior function to complete them, these typological unions often do not hold up in the long run. Eventually, what attracts partners to each other becomes what they despise if they do not develop some of these functions in themselves. So, the seeds of our potential undoing are sown right into the initial attraction.

Couples Therapy and Typology

As Jung notes and Wheelwright confirms,[62] one tends to be attracted to a person of the opposite typology because each partner is temporarily freed from the disagreeable task of dealing with their own inferior function.[63] Von Franz calls it "one of the great blessings and sources of happiness in the early stages of marriage; suddenly the whole of the inferior function is gone, one lives in a blessed oneness with the other, and every problem is solved!"[64] This is the oceanic feeling Freud describes where "at the height of being in love the boundary between ego and object threatens to melt away" and anyone in love who "declares that 'I' and 'you' are one behaves as if it were a fact."[65]

Couples typically do not seek therapy in the early honeymoon stage of relationship. They are still in their "blessed oneness," their own private

Garden of Eden, as it were. By the time couples do arrive in therapy, they are well past this stage. Judging by their levels of discontent and disdain, those oceanic feelings of blessed oneness are all but a distant memory. And like the consequences in the Garden, since it is impossible for couples to return to this early relationship stage, therapists are better served to help couples fully realize their current situation.

A couple's disillusionment can be explained and contextualized by highlighting their typological differences, providing a basis for deeper understanding and appreciation for one another. Unless addressed, typological differences will continue to affect relational dynamics and bolster archetypal deadlocks. For example, a thinker/feeler partnership may set up a parent/child dynamic, which, over time, constellates a *senex/puer* archetypal pair of opposites. Therapists can reframe these typological differences for couples as part of the individuation process within the relationship.

Clinically, typological problems are most evident when therapists see superior thinkers having little to no access to their inferior feeling function—just when they need it most—to connect with their superior feeling partners, and vice versa. As a clinician treating a couple with this typological constellation, notice how your own superior and inferior functions affect your countertransference. With whom do you find yourself aligning? Who do you find most frustrating?

Therapists should also be aware that patients can strongly prefer working with someone whose typology is opposite their own because the patient can "just sit there and hope that the other will do the work."[66] Accordingly, von Franz warns therapists to remain aware of their superior function and to use it with restraint. Even though it temporarily eases tensions, it also prevents the patient or a couple from doing the hard work of having to access their lesser conscious functions needed to solve their own problems. This would require, for example, a superior thinker to be more responsible for their own feelings and the superior feeler to take on a share of the thinking in the relationship, however difficult that may be for each of them.

With a couple's communication problems potentially rooted in typological differences, interrupting the flow of their conversation to highlight these differences can also be informative and enlightening. It can tease out what each partner is trying to communicate and what the other is missing due to typological differences. Consider the following vignette of a therapist working with a couple and their typological differences.

The Typical Typologist

Partner F (superior feeling function): [Loud, frustrated, angry.] *Every time you work late, it's like you don't care about me or the kids. I'm so sick of it! You never care about us. You always put yourself first. You never …*

Partner T (superior thinking function): [Interrupting, cool and calm, though with noticeable forced restraint.] *That's not true. I only worked late three times—three times, I counted them—over the past two weeks. Look at the calendar. See for yourself.*

Partner F (superior feeling function): [Heatedly.] *Oh God, here we go again. The stoic one with all the facts!*

Exasperated, both partners turn and glare at the therapist as if to say, *Do you see what I am dealing with here?*

Before continuing the dialogue, consider the impact of typological differences on this argument. In this classic and oversimplified example, thinkers always double down on facts and logic, while feelers double down on their feelings about what is happening. Therapists are tempted to align with one or the other depending on their own typology and will also feel frustrated by their typological opposite.

It can be hard for superior thinkers to give voice to their feelings.[67] Partner T does have feelings, but they are teeming in the unconscious and not readily accessible. Instead, Partner T has ready access to the data regarding the frequency of tardiness. Further, the superior thinking function often goes into overdrive in the face of rising emotion. Alternately, Partner F, the superior feeler, couldn't care less about what the *actual data* reveals and instead has ready access to the magnitude of the feeling of abandonment. Neither has access to their inferior function. The strong feeler cannot think clearly, and the strong thinker cannot find their feelings. As a result, the couple lacks empathy and understanding for each other. With whom should the therapist align? To which function should allegiance be pledged?

Many therapists who sense this all too familiar and uncomfortable trap attempt a way out by prescribing behavioral solutions. They might recommend Partner T call or text when they are going to be late or set definite times to be home. They might suggest that Partner T and Partner F track the number of late working days. While practical and helpful, the underlying issue—the intensity of their mutual frustration with each other—is left unaddressed. Therapists can extricate themselves from the referee position by assuming both partners are telling the truth, each from their own typological perspective. By highlighting a couple's typological differences in a non-pathologizing way, the therapist can offer a means of de-escalation and reconnection.

Continuing the dialogue, notice the therapist's empathy for both partners about how difficult this can be while inviting some access to their auxiliary functions:

Therapist: [Aware of their own typology and noticing with whom they are subtly—or not so subtly—aligning.] *OK, let's slow it down and pause a minute. Believe it or not, this has been helpful. I can see how frustrating this is for both of you. Let's go back and take it from the top. Partner F, can you repeat what you said about them working late? Go ahead, say it again.*

Partner F repeats the incident with heightened emotion and brings up another past incident that had caused distress. The therapist interrupts as quickly as possible.

Therapist: *OK, good. Let's hold it right there for now if you can. Now, Partner T: Can you repeat back, if you are able, what you just heard your partner tell you?*

Partner T (superior thinking function): *They said they are angry because they think I'm always late. But that's not true! The calendar shows ...*

Therapist: [Interrupting.] *Let's pause here for a moment. When passions are high, it is easy to forget what a strong thinker you are, Partner T, and what a strong feeler you are, Partner F. In these moments, we miss each other completely. [Turning to Partner F.] Partner F, your words come from a deep feeling place. Filtered through Partner T's strong thinking function, they get garbled. [Turning to Partner T.] Partner T, I see you trying to respond with your logical thinking words, which are getting misconstrued as they filter through Partner F's strong feeling function. [To both.] It's a wonder we ever communicate at all, given such big differences in how we experience each other and take in the world! One of you is a strong thinker, and the other a strong feeler. These opposites may be part of what attracted you to each other in the first place. It works well early in relationships, but the differences can become frustrating over time. The things we fall in love with about one another can become the things that drive us crazy later on unless we begin to do some work around them. Partner F, you are wanting your partner to feel a little more with you. Partner T, you are wanting your partner to be more rational and logical sometimes. Since neither of you can do this easily for one another, let's look at what you can do ...*

Ending the dialogue here, let us explore what can be done using the lens of typology. Since individuals have little access to their inferior function, it is often fruitless to demand information from it. Strong thinkers and feelers do, however, have conscious partial access to their auxiliary functions.[68] In this case, sensation and intuition may be partially available to both partners. After joining the strong thinker, using your own thinking function (if you have some access to it) and listening fully to what they *think* about the situation, ask them what their *intuition* tells them and what they *sense* about what is happening. Likewise, after using your feeling function (again, if you have access) to join with the strong feeler in bringing all their feelings to the forefront, ask them about their intuitions and sense impressions.

Let the couple know what you are doing and why. As they find some common ground and mutual empathy again through their auxiliary functions, invite the couple to practice the same approach whenever they find themselves at odds. That is, share from the superior function, but more importantly, explore more fully through auxiliary functions to help stay connected. For some couples, these auxiliary functions may also be at odds, but the shift away from their usual entrenchment and warring narrative may open space for further nuance and curiosity about one's self and the other.[69] Either way, interrupting the flow of heated conversation is difficult to do in real time. For a fuller exploration of facilitating couple's dialogues, see the work of Joan Pieniadz and Polly Young-Eisendrath.[70]

Returning to the dialogue above, on the surface, nothing appears to have been resolved. However, the therapist has extricated themself, for the time being, from the judge-and-jury power position.[71]

If the couple faces a longstanding problem (or one that keeps showing up in different guises), it is usually a sign that their superior functions are of little use in resolving this kind of issue. The inferior function could easily settle it, but the partners have no conscious access to it. Therefore, the auxiliary functions are needed to help tackle the problem. For example, therapists can invite superior thinkers to pay close attention to what their intuition and sense impressions tell them. They may then be able to make some headway in uncertain territory where their feeling function could have easily shown the way.

Conclusion

This chapter has briefly explored the *conscious* aspects of Jung's typological theory and introduced its use in couples therapy. In an age of positivism, behavioral training, and manualized approaches, it can feel uncomfortable to accept that we have an innate temperament and that our typology (notwithstanding some normal fluctuations in life) is, well, kind of what it is. We all have an inferior function and, with it, our shortcomings and blind spots. No matter how hard a superior thinker tries, they will never have a superior feeling function, for "nothing disturbs thinking so much as feeling, and the feeling type represses thinking, since nothing is more injurious to feeling than thinking."[72] However, all is not lost. There is partial conscious access to the auxiliary functions, and since they do not pose a major threat to the superior function, partners can use them to connect, if possible.

Do not underestimate the impact that fundamental typological differences have on relationships. These differences have the power to cast love spells and to disenchant. They can often be at the root of the intractable problems that couples bring to therapy. Once brought to consciousness, working with typology can be an easy, powerful, and rewarding way to help individuals in relationship distinguish themselves from one another.

Jung's complete theory of typology is multifaceted and complex. For example, it also accounts for the compensatory relationship between the conscious and unconscious whereby one's conscious typology functions simultaneously in an opposite way in the unconscious.[73] Thus, a conscious extraversion is compensated for by an unconscious introverted egocentrism. Jung says that if left unacknowledged, it will remain regressive and will show itself in infantile behavior when it erupts into consciousness.

Even at an introductory level, therapists familiar with the basics of typology can establish a framework for couples to begin to consciously acknowledge their often profound differences in ways that do not feel blaming, threatening, pathologizing, or abandoning. When therapists highlight and de-pathologize basic typological differences, couples often report having more empathy for one another and themselves. Some couples even begin to appreciate, support, and feel protective of these differences. We encourage you to invite couples to review the tables in this chapter and then explore how they see themselves and each other. Help them imagine into their superior and inferior functions and name and use their auxiliary functions to build a bridge back to one another. Even with that bridging, however, all our typological differences ultimately (and sadly) mean, *no one is like you.* While this frustrates the desire for deep connection through sameness, it can lead to celebration of difference, an altogether distinct and fruitful path toward intimacy.

Notes

1 Jung 1971[1921], p. xi.
2 Jung 1963, p. 207.
3 Even the popular Enneagram Personality Test, while not based upon Jung's typology, is based upon his theories of the archetypes and the complex.
4 Some of the nuance in Jung's typological theory is sacrificed for ease of use with the Myers-Briggs Type Indicator (Karesh et al. 1994), while the less well-known Singer-Loomis Type Deployment Inventory may retain more of its original complexity (Spoto 1995).
5 Harrell 2017.
6 Beebe 2017.
7 Sharp 1987.
8 Spoto 1995.
9 von Franz & Hillman 1971.
10 Wheelwright 1982.
11 Jung 1971[1921], para. 687.
12 Jung 1971[1921], para. 690.
13 Sharp 1991, p. 52.
14 Spoto 1995.
15 Jung 1989.
16 Spoto 1995.
17 Sharp 1991, p. 75.
18 Wheelwright 1982.
19 Jung 1971[1921], paras 577–665.
20 Beebe 2017, p. 147.
21 Beebe 2017, p. 147.
22 Beebe 2017, p. 147.
23 Sharp 1987, p.17.
24 Jung 1971[1921], para. 774.
25 Jung 1971[1921], para. 792.
26 Jung 1989.
27 Spoto 1995, p. 46.
28 Jung 1971[1921], para. 830.
29 Spoto 1995, p. 45.
30 Jung 1971[1921].
31 von Franz 2008[1986], p. 16.
32 Jung 1971[1921], para. 770.
33 Jung 1931, para. 955.
34 Jung 1971[1921].

35 Sharp 1987.
36 Corrie 2015[1927].
37 Corrie 2015[1927].
38 Jung 1971[1921].
39 Corrie 2015[1927], p. 38.
40 Jung 1989.
41 Corrie 2015[1927].
42 Jung 1971[1921].
43 Jung 1971[1921].
44 Beebe 2017.
45 Jung 1971[1921].
46 Jung 1971[1921].
47 Sharp 1987.
48 Jung 1971[1921], para. 640.
49 Corrie 2015[1927].
50 Jung 1971[1921].
51 Corrie 2015[1927].
52 Corrie 2015[1927], para. 613.
53 Beebe 2017, p. 5.
54 Jung, 1971[1921].
55 Sharp 1987.
56 Jung 1971[1921], para. 654.
57 Sharp 1987.
58 Jung 1971[1921].
59 Jung 1953, para. 85.
60 von Franz & Hillman 1971, p. 59.
61 Jung 1953, para. 85.
62 Wheelwright 1982.
63 von Franz & Hillman 1971, p. 59.
64 von Franz & Hillman 1971, p. 59, p. 4.
65 Freud 1930, p. 66.
66 von Franz & Hillman 1971, pp. 4–5.
67 Jung 1931.
68 Jung 1971[1921].
69 John Beebe (2017) notes that our lesser conscious parenting and inner child arche-types, both their positive and shadowed aspects, are found in these auxiliary functions.
70 Pieniadz & Young-Eisendrath 2021.
71 For those familiar with Melanie Klein's (1946) foundational psychoanalytic for-mulation, the partners have been invited to move from their split paranoid-schizoid (PS) position back to the depressive (D) position, where they are able to process more of what is happening through their auxiliary functions, tolerate more distress resulting from their typological differences, and mourn the loss of the illusion of their once-idealized partner.
72 Jung 1923, para. 905.
73 Jung 1971[1921].

References

Beebe, J. (2017). *Energies and patterns in psychological type*. Routledge.
Corrie, J. (2015). *ABC of Jung's psychology*. Routledge. (Original work published 1927.)
Freud, S. (1930). Civilization and its discontents. *SE* XXI.

Harrell, E. (2017). A brief history of personality tests. *Harvard Business Review*, 95(2), 63.

Jung, C. G. (1923). Psychological types. *CW* 6.

Jung, C. G. (1931). *A psychological theory of types. CW* 6.

Jung, C. G.(1953). Two essays on analytical psychology. *CW* 7.

Jung, C. G. (1963). *Memories, dreams, reflections* (A. Jaffé, Ed.; R. Winston & C. Winston, Trans.; Rev. ed.). Vintage. (Original work published 1961.)

Jung, C. G. (1971). Psychological types. *CW* 6. (Original work published 1921.)

Jung, C. G. (1989). *Analytical psychology, notes of the seminar given in 1925 by C. G. Jung* (W. McGuire, Ed.). Princeton University Press.

Karesh, D. M., Pieper, W. A., & Holland, C. L. (1994). Comparing the MBTI, the Jungian type survey, and the Singer-Loomis inventory of personality. *Journal of Psychological Types*, 30, 30–38.

Klein, M. (1946). Notes on some schizoid mechanisms. *International Journal of Psycho-analysis*, 27, 99–110.

Pieniadz, J., & Young-Eisendrath, P. (2021). *Dialogue therapy for couples and real dialogue for opposing sides.* Routledge.

Sharp, D. (1987). *Personality types.* Inner City.

Sharp, D.(1991). *C. G. Jung lexicon.* Inner City.

Spoto, A. (1995). *Jung's typology in perspective* (Rev. ed.). Chiron.

von Franz, M-L. (2008). C. G. Jung's rehabilitation of the feeling function in our civilization. *Jung Journal*, 2(2), 9–20. (Original work published 1986.)

von Franz, M-L., & Hillman, J. (1971). *Jung's typology.* Spring.

Wheelwright, J. B. (1982). *Saint George and the dandelion.* C.G. Jung Institute of San Francisco.

Chapter 5

The Shadow and the Couple[1]

Around the time C. G. Jung began to intellectually differentiate himself from Sigmund Freud—a deeply painful rupture for both men—he had an important dream. In the dream, Jung carries a small lamp that illuminates his person and casts a large, hulking shadow into the darkness behind him. As with so many dreams, Jung viewed it as the psyche speaking in its native language: image. The dream contrasts the light of consciousness with the inevitability of shadow of unconsciousness. Jung defines the shadow as all the things we cannot perceive and do not want to accept about ourselves, often aspects of our character we deny, ignore, or repress. Yet the shadow constantly accompanies us; it is us. Ironically, the place where we aspire to be our best selves, committed relationships, is precisely where our shadow is most frequently revealed. These are the aspects couples bring to therapy for treatment.

Everybody—that is every *body*—casts a shadow. For Jungians, self-knowledge requires courageous confrontation with the shadow. Shadow work is motivated by the desire to know oneself in depth, and it is an important part of the individuation process. Freud likewise emphasized the importance of self-knowledge. The fundamental premise of psychoanalysis, he asserts, is recognition that "the psychical" includes both consciousness and unconsciousness.[2]

In the last century, Freud's desire to make the unconscious conscious became the cornerstone of psychoanalysis.[3] The existence of unconsciousness slowly pervaded other forms of psychotherapy, whether the Freudian influence was acknowledged or not. Even behavior modification therapies require patients to become more conscious of their actions before change can take place. In addition to rooting out causes in an unconscious past, Jung asserts that the unconscious is also forward-looking; its processes are dynamic and continuously creative. Therapists look to the unconscious not only for past causes to current troubles, but also for what is emerging now and wants to emerge in the near future.

The psyche actively participates in the individuation of the partners and the individuation of the relationship through bringing unconscious tensions to the surface. It is as if the promise to love, honor, and cherish one's partner is destined to introduce (or induce) their opposites, including impatience, resentment, and discontent. Over time, therapists and their couples learn to

DOI: 10.4324/9781032688008-6

tolerate such tensions as inevitable, even necessary, as they make their way through dark nights of the soul together, relying on the lamp of insight, or inner sight, for guidance while simultaneously remaining aware of the shadow cast behind.

Jung's concept of the shadow has become part of the lexicon of psychotherapists working in many traditions probably because it is such a sensible, practical idea. It is "the image of ourselves that slides along behind us as we walk toward the light," says Murray Stein.[4] The twin idea, the persona, which "is the face we wear to meet the social world around us,"[5] is similarly sensible and practical. Together, shadow and persona shape a more rounded sense of identity and individuality. Robert Johnson describes the shadow as "a curious dark element that follows us like a saurian tail," the part of us "we fail to see and know."[6] He contrasts it with the persona, which is "what we would like to be and how we wish to be seen by the world."[7] Robert Bly describes the shadow as the long bag we drag behind us, which we steadily fill with all of the things that parents, teachers, and peers tell us *not* to be. "We spend our life until we are twenty deciding what parts of ourself to put into the bag," says Bly, "and we spend the rest of our lives trying to get them back out again."[8]

"The construction of a collectively suitable persona means a formidable concession to the external world," Jung admits, "a genuine self-sacrifice which drives the ego straight into identification with the persona, so that people do really exist who believe they are what they pretend to be."[9] The shadow, as a result, "personifies everything that the subject refuses to acknowledge about himself and yet is always thrusting itself upon him directly or indirectly."[10] No matter how much one attempts to ignore or repress one's shadow, the effort will fail. Jung points out that the contents of the shadow are not necessarily negative. They are "merely somewhat inferior, primitive, unadapted, and awkward" and contain qualities that "vitalize and embellish human existence, but convention forbids!"[11] For those who have negative beliefs about themselves, the shadow will contain all their positive attributes they have disavowed.

Shadow, Persona, and the Couple

Shadow and persona dance together in social life for all of us, to be sure, but the pressure on couples is particularly intense. Many people, not just the partners, are invested in a couple's happily-ever after persona because it symbolizes persistent cultural fantasies about finding *the one* and living together in domestic harmony. Pressure to maintain the illusion of being a happy couple can make the partners' suffering especially poignant since another cultural fantasy—sometimes a reality—is that intimate relationships are the refuge where truth, no matter how shameful, can be spoken. Most people long to admit secret desires, dreams, and failings in intimate relationships and hope that the one they love will greet their whole self with compassion and acceptance. But it is complicated. As Jung intimates, people generally want to believe they are who they think they are, usually some version of their idealized self, which makes acknowledging the existence of a shadow, let alone accepting its contents, difficult indeed.[12]

Jung describes confronting the shadow as the apprentice-piece of individuation and the first obstacle in the journey towards wholeness.[13] It often begins when the idealized persona has grown brittle, and is seen for what it is: a mask that disguises aspects of character the person rejects or considers unacceptable—even, in some instances, unthinkable. Intimate partners, for instance, discover they can be angry, nasty, and unkind to the one they love—altogether without the endless compassion and generosity they vowed to sustain in the relationship. Or, for instance, therapists discover their own incapacities and limitations, not their skillfulness, despite all their years of training and all their accumulated experience and knowledge. The shadow of therapeutic expertise shows up in moments when they have no idea what to say to a couple sitting a few feet away who is enraged, in tears, or stonily silent, and simply being with them in the emotional chaos or despair feels wholly inadequate.

Jungian theory of the persona and shadow reveals unconscious identity conflicts *within* partners. Each person confronts the internal tension between the roles they learn to play, a social self that is rarely questioned, and an original self, that "deep and eternal person" who exists "far beneath the many thick layers of indoctrination about who we are and who we should be."[14] The multiple personae that comprise a social presence in the world are useful and necessary adaptations so long as people do not confuse them with the entirety of who they are.

Couples, whether married or not, often have vivid associations to the labels *wife* and *husband*. These associations change with the times, of course, and differ from culture to culture. But some associations have persisted for centuries, including the idea that *the wife* is devoted to the private, domestic sphere of home and children, a natural caregiver, while *the husband* bravely ventures into the public world as the provider. When the associations to these labels are mostly positive, people are eager to marry. When mostly negative, they may reject marriage but, in some cases, still desire intimacy with another. In either case, an emotional response to the labels *wife* and *husband* indicates how strongly role expectations influence the partners' image of themselves in a relationship, what they expect of the other, and how such expectations shape the rhythms of coupled life. With the creation of these idealized personae, much is relegated to the shadow. Striving to be ideal instead of real causes intrapsychic tension between partners.

Individual Shadows in Relationship

Emotionally committed relationships offer an incomparable opportunity for each partner to confront their personal shadow. For example, Jungian analyst

Marion Woodman describes her decades-long marriage as a "precious gift" that "burned away the dross and left the gold,"[15] a fiery image that alludes to the intense heat of intimacy. Their relationship kept Woodman and her husband "dancing in the flames," the title of one of her books,[16] taken from a Zen koan.

What types of dross get burned away in the heat of committed relationship? One kind is the persona partners develop in their youth, which persist into adulthood with surprising tenacity. The persona, and its accompanying shadow, can often be generated early in the family of origin. Consider, for instance, the labels siblings are given as children: the serious one, the funny one, the brave one, the smart one, the flighty one, the athletic one, and so on. Children quickly catch on to the idea implicit in the label itself: there can be only *one* of each. They learn to divide roles partly to gain attention and partly to avoid conflict with others. A problem arises when children over-identify with these labels and continue to believe that the label defines them as they grow up, which creates their shadow. For example, the serious one's playful side is relegated to the shadows of the unconscious, or the athletic one disavows their intelligence.

Unless worked through, these personae and their assigned role designations continue to influence adult relationships. Therapists can ask partners about them: *How were you labeled as a child? Do those labels still work for you today? What else is also true about you? What roles are you playing in your relationship? Which ones still work, and which ones have become constraining? If you could let go of those roles, even just a little, how might that be for you and your partner? Let's ask your partner how they might feel about it ...*

As therapists help partners clarify the personae they regularly use with one another, often unconsciously, the work will simultaneously reveal what they hide in their shadow, and how both persona and shadow impact relationship dynamics. Such self-knowledge expands each partner's psychological world, including both the sense of themselves within the relationship as well as their sense of self beyond it. Raising these things to awareness with couples can increase tension, both inter-psychically and intra-psychically, but one of Jung's core insights is that conflict "stirs consciousness."[17] Conflict, the thing most people are taught to limit or avoid, is the soul's way of inciting (and inviting) individuation. Over time, therapists learn to be more comfortable with this type of discomfort.

Shadow Work and the Culture of the Relationship

Bly makes an important point about the long bag of shadow material we drag behind us, mentioned above. "Different cultures fill the bag with different contents."[18] He affirms Jung's point that *convention* forbids specific beliefs and behaviors. The different cultures Bly mentions refer to the microculture of one's own family, the larger society and historical era that shape a generation, and the various religious, political, and gender identities (among other kinds of identity) that intersect to comprise the complex people we are. Many couples may not imagine tension in their relationship as a cultural conflict, yet Jung's expanded notion of the Self as individual and collective (see Chapter 1) suggests it is so. Partners bring the microculture of their family of origin as well as intergenerational assumptions, beliefs, and wounds that cohere in patterns of relating. Such patterns remain largely unconscious until they erupt.

The therapeutic encounter becomes a multi-cultural space where the worlds and worldviews of partners can surface as part of the journey towards self-knowledge. Of course, therapists must remain aware, to the degree they are able, of how their own worldview and cultural background influence the space. Partners often fall unconsciously into patterns of thought and behavior that bear an uncanny resemblance to their parent's behavior—or the opposite, as compensation. Such patterns arise from ethnic, religious, class, political, and cultural indoctrination regardless of whether they collide with hard-earned personal values. When partners grow up in dissimilar cultures, their differences are usually apparent. When partners grow up in the same culture, it may be more difficult to recognize divergent beliefs and assumptions about intimate relationship. One such difference might be as simple and as powerful as each person's associations to silence. *When my partner is quiet, she's really angry with me*, assumes one person. But that may not be true at all. They may just enjoy a quiet home.

In either case, partners unconsciously try to recreate the culture of their family of origin and have little or no idea of its effects on the relationship. Shadow work may begin with tender examination of each partner's inherited customs and beliefs, exploring what aligns with their values and discarding what does not (or trying to; inherited patterns are tenacious). Shadow work also can include finer differentiation of *this is me, this is you*, with a sense of appreciation, mutual respect, and even playfulness. In the end, what felt like a *collision* of worlds—cultural, religious, ethnic, political, and other differences—can become a kind of *meeting* of worlds characterized by empathy and acceptance. Ideally, it becomes the foundation of greater soulfulness for both partners.

Confronting the Shadow in the Context of Relationship

Conflict between partners usually indicates movement toward a more psychological relationship. This arduous and ongoing process toward greater consciousness requires partners to deal with their emerging shadow material. Recalling Woodman's image, couples must be able to dance in the flames of growing awareness *together*.

There is a particular poignance and intensity to shadow work in relationship. It is less private and more relentless than individual shadow work since the relationship holds up a mirror in which the partners see themselves. As Jung says, deep understanding of the shadow is impossible without a human partner, since confessing it to another makes it all very real.

A general and merely academic "insight into one's mistakes" is ineffectual, for then the mistakes are not really seen at all, only the idea of them. But they show up acutely when a human relationship brings them to the fore and when they are noticed by the other person as well as by oneself. Then and only then can they really be felt and their true nature recognized. Similarly, confessions made to one's secret self generally have little or no effect, whereas confessions made to another are much more promising.[19]

Exploring the shadow in therapy challenges the partners to reveal more of their whole selves with the person they love, even when trust has broken down or when they are unsure of, or ambivalent about, the relationship's future. The risks are great, without question, but the rewards of discovering a more soulful relationship together are greater.

Shadow work may be a couple's first step into the unconscious with their chosen partner, and the learning curve is sometimes precipitous. It often produces a surprising and disorienting loss of a familiar identity owing to naïve confidence in the completeness of one's own self-knowledge. Realizing the existence of the shadow is a *symbolic* death because a couple's ideas of who they think they are dissolves. Mythically, confrontation with the shadow can be compared to descent into the underworld, the direction of soul travel as Heraclitus intimates in one of his more famous fragments: "You could not discover the limits of soul, even if you traveled every road to do so; such is the depth of its meaning."[20]

If working with shadow is an apprenticeship, the archetypal question becomes, *Who is the teacher?* There are many possible answers to this question, but one that may suffice for a suffering couple is: *the relationship.* That is, the relationship itself calls partners to discover the limits of their own souls and the soul of their union. The union invites them down into the underworld of what they do not yet know and yet is necessary for their individuation. As discussed in Chapter 3, some of the most beloved and retold myths of descent into the underworld, from Sumerian, Egyptian, Greek and Roman sources, feature marriage—and an encounter with death.

Excursion: Psyche, Eros, and the Necessity of Death

When couples engage in a psychological relationship, they die symbolically, numerous times. The 2,000-year-old story about the marriage of Eros (Amor) and the Soul (Psyche) is an interesting case study illustrating the death motif in coupled life.

In the tale, Psyche is the youngest daughter of the King and Queen, so lovely that the community regards her as a fresh incarnation of Aphrodite, the goddess of Love and Beauty. Naturally, this enrages the goddess. Psyche is also fated to marry a monster, sometimes described as Death itself. Her family bows to fate. Psyche's parents arrange a wedding in which the procession of the bride towards the altar is a funeral march. They abandon Psyche at the edge of cliff and turn away, fully expecting her to die. Instead, Aphrodite's boyish son, Eros, falls in love with Psyche and carries her off to his golden palace, where the lovers live in clandestine bliss for a short time.

Three moments from the story illustrate the death motif present in soulful relationships. First, Psyche is suicidal after Eros abandons her and nearly succeeds in drowning herself in the river. Second, Psyche endures the killing rage of Aphrodite, who gives the young woman four impossible tasks she is never meant to survive. Third, Psyche fails to complete the fourth and final task—a journey to the realm of the Dead—and falls into a death-like trance. In the end, Psyche prevails in part because she has demonstrated fidelity to Eros and has faced death repeatedly. Each symbolic death is a transformative threshold that draws her toward new life.[21]

Couples appearing for therapy may very well be in the midst of psychological death. Something has prompted them to try therapy, possibly a deep, unconscious desire to create a more soulful relationship. As the story of Eros and Psyche illustrates, the journey is long and difficult. Many things must symbolically die on the way, including fantasies about what life as a couple should be like. Another is the fantasy of *who I will be as a partner*, those stereotyped thoughts and behavior patterns that partners imagine (or hope) they can sustain. A third kind of fantasy is how my partner will treat me, *how I will be loved, how my wounds will be healed*. Such fantasies are the legacy of relational assumptions and patterns developed early in life, discussed earlier. They are also fed by culturally transmitted forms of knowledge from books, cinema, or news media that portray happy or successful couples or the inverse, bitter and embattled couples.

Fantasies of coupled life are not in themselves bad or destructive. They reflect imaginative engagement with one's partner and with the idea of partnership, which can nourish coupled life and inspire loving behavior. However, when the fantasies become coercive scripts propping up the idea of being a perfect partner or perfect couple, they are damaging. On this topic, Jung's comment on perfection is a suitable warning. He says there is "considerable difference between *perfection* and *completeness.*"[22] There may be perfection in striving for completeness (wholeness), but there is never wholeness in perfection. Partners who psychologically carve themselves into an acceptable form to be perfect by rejecting qualities that do not fit their ideal cannot face their shadow. *Sugar and spice and everything nice, that's what little girls are made of*, goes the nineteenth century nursery rhyme. Although this prescription may appear 200 years out of date, it has remarkable persistence as an unconscious psychological script.

Vows and Shadow Vows

Wedding vows express many fantasies of ideal or perfect coupling. The public nature of ceremonies often induces couples to present perfect selves to each other and, sometimes, to create the illusion of a perfect couple, much to the envy of friends or family unable to see below the surface. But it does not have to be that way. Instead, partners can begin creating a psychological relationship from the outset by composing vows that encompass more of the totality of the Self, including their shadowed selves.

Solemn vows are sacred, carrying deep and private meaning for the two persons. Thus, although weddings are public rituals, only a couple knows what has moved in their souls. And they do not know where that movement may take them. The mystery of relationship, one that can only be lived, makes the shadowy counterpart of every loving vow painful to confront. Yet every spoken vow has its accompanying shadow, comprised of all that remained unspoken and unconscious when the partners say, *I do*. These shadow vows are the unacknowledged assumptions, agreements, and obligations each partner brings to the relationship.

When vows are spoken, the evocative archetypal patterns of *husband* and *wife* are now constellated in the relationship—even for same-sex couples in which gay men refer to their partner as *my husband* or lesbians speak of their partner as *my wife*. This archetypal shift often predates the exchange of vows as couples imagine into married life. *What will it be like to be a husband?* Or *What kind of wife will I be?* For each partner the role designations come loaded with assumptions, fantasies, and desires, which are rarely conscious. That is, *husband* and *wife* have large shadows. Therapists might notice the presence of shadow material when partners stop using each other's name in complaints such as, *I just want a wife who's glad to see me when I come home*, or *I need a husband who's going to step up and be there for me*. Helping couples distinguish their role expectations from the flesh-and-blood person they married is difficult.

The conscious vow, as emissary, is always accompanied by a shadowed twin. Both are messengers, ever revealing more of ourselves to ourselves—and to our partner. Although mutual vulnerability is one of love's great gifts, it is never easy. In fact, vulnerability is "infinitely more demanding than the effort we put into avoidance of intimacy."[23] Revelation consists of "giving the other sufficient emotional space in which to live and express her soul, with its reasonable and unreasonable ways, and then to risk revealing your own soul, complete with its own absurdities."[24] Such revelation is only possible when the relationship is sturdy enough to withstand confrontation with the shadow. By its very nature, the act of coming to therapy together (and surviving it) can sometimes strengthen the relational container.

A Jungian approach with couples reimagines their troubles as the soul speaking, not as moral or spiritual failure. The relationship may be most soulful when it is most troubled, a unique and incomparable vale of soul-making. Few other experiences, except parenting, come close because relationships land couples exactly in the chaos of old wounds, and it does not cure them. Discord, when seen as a *via regia* to the soul of a relationship, is trying to reveal what the soul needs. Partners can explore uncomfortable questions such as, *How does this conflict show me a shadow vow? How does it*

unveil, albeit painfully perhaps, a fuller truth about a promise I made to myself,
my partner, or my relationship?

In addition to *shadow vows*, there are other evocative descriptions of this
phenomenon. Mythopoeist Robert Bly, for instance, says that when a couple
exchanges conscious vows, they simultaneously and unconsciously exchange a
set of private vows in the basement below the altar.[25] Psychoanalyst Judith
Pickering uses the phrase *malignant dowry* to describe the "encrypted pattern
of engagement that each partner brings" to the relationship, contributing to
"extremely complex and entangled" dramas.[26] James Hollis says the public
ceremony is haunted by another drama unfolding in the shadows.[27] There is a
subtle suggestion in some of this language that exchanging vows is a Janus-
faced performance art, one intended for the public and the other private, one
in the light, the other unconsciously enacted in the shadows.

Even when couples have decided against civil or religious ceremonies, they
are still subjected to the shadowed aspects of commitment. In such cases the
language of dowry or vow does not fully suit the situation, yet they still laugh
knowingly at the pithy definition of shadow vows: *What we don't say when we*
say, "I do." In fact, many partners who choose not to marry may have
exchanged spoken vows in their own unique commitment ceremony. Many
also make commitments to themselves about who they want to be in a relationship. An honest discussion between the partners in the context of therapy
can bring to light both spoken and unspoken promises they live each day.
Such commitments are revealed in word, posture, gesture, and action.

Excursion: Playing in the Shadows

Many decades ago, the American Conservatory Theater (ACT) in San Francisco
created an extraordinary rendition of Shakespeare's tale of love and hatred *The*
Taming of the Shrew. The play is justly criticized for its overt misogyny, yet ACT's
fresh interpretation dramatized a profound psychological truth summed up in Jung's
statement "hatred is tremendous cement."[28]

When the curtain opened, audiences were treated to a stark set design that
immediately suggested two concurrent narratives, one in the limelight and the other
in the shadows. Centered on the stage was a large raised square platform, a stage
within the stage, framed on three sides with vertical wooden studs eighteen inches
apart to suggest walls, like the framing of a half-built house. As some readers know,
the so-called courtship of the main characters, Petruchio and Katherina, more closely resembles martial conquest; Petruchio's methods of taming the shrew of the
play's title are truly cruel; he seems to relish tormenting her. In ACT's performance,
each of the couple's battles were played out on the well-lit raised platform. Immediately after their scenes together, the actors quickly separated like a pair of prize
fighters (which they were, in some sense), strode around the side walls and eagerly
re-met at the center back of the stage in a passionate embrace. If this was acting,

the audience was utterly convinced. The emotional complexity the director and the players so brilliantly conveyed was simply unforgettable.

The performance was a dramatic reminder that even at the pitch of intimate battle, there is always more going on between couples than meets the eye. When couples fight, therapists can ask partners how or why expressing their frustration, anger, rage, and yes, even hatred, serves to keep them entwined.

Speech of the Soul and Wisdom of the Body

When sitting with couples, it is difficult to create enough space to allow partners to explore the fullness of what is going on beneath their anger or frustrations. A significant amount of time can be spent listening to couples vent and indict one another, rather than thinking about and working on their issues. Sometimes, it takes tremendous effort just to slow couples down in sessions. If and when they are able to re-regulate themselves, it also takes time to craft a reliably safe space for both partners (if it is available between them) to find the speech of the heart and soul that expresses their deepest wounds and longings.

Slowing down the dialog between partners also encourages deeply buried somatic knowledge to present itself, which often needs to be invited to the surface of consciousness. The body expresses the truth, even when the mind resists, though this is a fact few people, even experts in the healing professions, acknowledge. Jung was a pioneer in this regard. In his essay "The Spiritual Problem of Modern Man" he says:

> The mysterious truth is that the spirit is the life of the body seen from within, and the body is the outward manifestation of the life of the spirit—the two being really one. Striving to transcend the present level of consciousness through the acceptance of the unconscious must give the body its due.[29]

Acknowledging the wisdom of the body, long expressed in the work of somatic pioneers such as Wilhelm Reich and Alexander Lowen,[30] has been confirmed by contemporary neuroscience and features prominently in therapeutic approaches to trauma. It is captured in the title of Bessel van der Kolk's 2015 book, *The Body Keeps the Score.*

Making room for the truth of the body is a significant psychological achievement for both couple and therapist. Finding a fit between somatic experience and verbal language is equally significant. When a true statement is vocalized, the result is somatic release. The patient often sighs or exhales, or their shoulders soften, the jaw unclenches, and the face relaxes. Attuning to somatic cues helps couples pay attention to their embodied experience together as another expression of the soul of the relationship.

The Paradoxical and Contradictory Nature of Commitment

Recall that the aim of psychological relationship is wholeness, which means everything belongs—including the shadow qualities partners want to disavow. Consciously or unconsciously, couples bring their best *and* worst selves to the relationship. Voicing shadow vows frequently requires partners to accept and embody emotional paradox, feelings that contradict one another. For example, *I like being together, but sometimes I wish I were still single.* Or, *My partner is kind and loving, but they drive me crazy at times.* For some couples, the mere thought of having such mixed or ambivalent emotions is threatening. It can feel like both a moral failure and a personal one. Therapists help couples normalize the paradoxical feelings found in all relationships by encouraging the addition of time-limiting words. For example, *I love my partner but* right now *I don't like them very much.*

In addition to having contradictory emotions, shadow content may show when a partner has two needs that are incompatible with one another. For example, *I love living with you, but I also need time alone.* Or, *I enjoy having sex with you, but there are times when I am not in the mood.* Such needs can be especially problematic if they compete with established ideas of how loving partners *should* be in a relationship. If the incompatible needs persist, it may be an intense desire of the soul necessary for individuation. As frustration rises, conflict becomes unavoidable. Naming these needs often creates uneasiness because partners risk being seen as the whole people they are, with all their deeply human needs, inconsistencies, and conflicting desires. As mentioned earlier, it takes immense courage to be honest with oneself and vulnerable with one another. The phrase *shadow vow* captures the vivid emotional and somatic truth of this challenge. Eventually, couples who work through the shadowed aspects of their vows can tolerate these contradictions and slowly develop the capacity for seeing through discord to its deeper meanings. It is ongoing work, as Jung insists. The shadow accompanies us everywhere, all the time. We *never* master or eradicate it. The moment we think we have, we get into trouble.

Most people do not make commitments lightly. But even thoughtful, serious people may not fully come to terms with how competing commitments—what poet David Whyte refers to as *metaphorical marriages*—create tension in relationships.[31] Yet the idea of metaphorical marriage is found in everyday language when, for example, people speak about *being married to my job.* Therapists can help couples notice how these other commitments impact their relationship. These commitments are often profound and lifelong, and viewing them as metaphorical marriages grants them the status they may deserve. This helps couples more clearly see and negotiate their needs. What takes precedence—home, family and friends, work, community, a cause, or the creative life—shows how someone invests their time, the most precious form of wealth any of us has. Once each partner names their meaningful commitments, therapists can help them explore their impact on the relationship.

When one partner needs to devote hours to writing a novel, training for a marathon, or playing golf on Saturday morning, the nourishment they gain from it might ease tensions in the relationship—if their partner can tolerate or even support their absence. That competing demand may well be a necessity, part of their soul work, and the psyche can be quite ruthless in its demands. Therapists might ask couples (and themselves), *With such passion for these other commitments, what implicit vows have you made to your own soul? How do you live out those vows?* Asking both partners, *What impact do you think this is having on your relationship? In what ways do you feel torn or supported or abandoned?* Such questions are true to Jung's definition of individuation as a dynamic, unending transformative process—a sacred endeavor centered on the realization of the fuller Self, not the ego.

Helping couples recognize their metaphorical marriages, and give voice to their vows and shadow vows, can usher in the proper ending to their outworn fantasies of an ideal relationship. Doing so can make way for a symbolic second relationship between the same two people, when something truer and more authentic grows in its place. On the other hand, voicing shadow vows can bring insurmountable troubles to the surface, signaling a need to separate or divorce. Regardless of the outcome, a couple's willingness to explore shadow vows is soul work, part of the life of the relationship that "wants to be loved, to be heard, to be named and seen."[32]

Couples in Conflict and Jung's Quaternity

Figure 5.1 is a variation of Jung's quaternity diagram, which he introduced in an essay on the mutual transformation of the therapist and patient in clinical work.[33] It can also be used to depict the psychological dynamics at play between two partners in relationship.

In Figure 5.1, the upper a-line represents the conscious relationship between partners. The b-lines represent each partner's relationship to their unconscious.

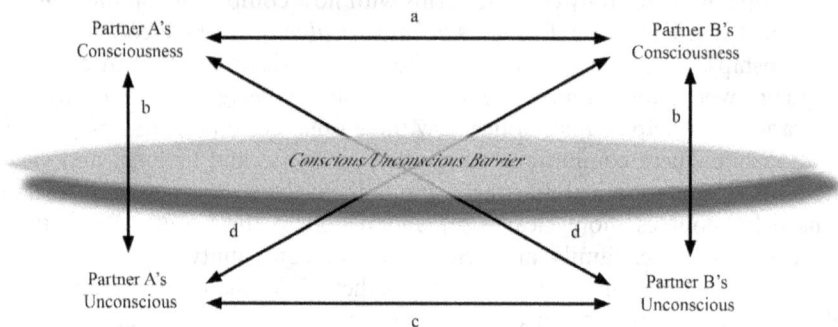

Figure 5.1 Variation on Jung's Quaternity. From "The Psychology of the Transference" (para. 422) in *CW* 16, by C. G. Jung, 1946. Princeton University Press. Adapted with permission.

The lower c-line represents the unconscious relationship between the partners. The crossing d-lines highlight the conscious and unconscious projections made by each partner onto the other. The quaternity diagram is useful because it illustrates the complicated psychic field in which couples therapy takes place. By considering these lines of influence, therapists can use the diagram to orient themselves to the unconscious origins of some of the persistent distress between the partners.

For the purposes of couples therapy, the upper a-line represents the partners' conscious vows or commitments to one another. The lower c-line, which depicts the unconscious-to-unconscious relationship between partners, is the unknown region of shadow vows and, eventually, the place from which they rise into consciousness. Vertical b-lines depict the intrapsychic relationship of each partner to their inner world, partly conscious and partly unconscious, as indicated by the barrier in Figure 5.1. The diagonal d-lines are the conscious and unconscious values, needs, and demands that the partners project onto/into each other.

The b- and d-line dynamics often show up overtly in therapy as the stress points for couples. They present a creative opportunity for insight into the soul of both partners and the soul of their relationship. Initially, therapists meet couples right where they are, by working with their most conscious material represented by the quaternity's a-line. By inviting partners to recall their original vows to one another, and how they have lived these vows, they reveal the emotional complexity of lifelong commitment. For example, as partners reconsider their vow to love and honor, the question can be asked, *In what ways have I also felt hatred or disrespect for my partner?*

The c-line dynamic, the least accessible psychological content and the deepest source of shadow vows, may not show up overtly but emerges through the exploration of b- and d-line tensions. Working with unconscious material along any of these vectors is reclamation in the truest sense. It invites each partner to take back what is emotionally theirs and allows them to see themselves and each other more fully.

Shadow Themes in Therapy

As mentioned in Chapter 1, research has shown that, on average, couples are six years late in coming to therapy.[34] The enactment of shadow vows often emerges slowly over the years because couples attempt to keep the peace through conflict avoidance, repression, silence, rationalization, and cognitive reframing. When couples' dynamics include hatred, abandonment, or selfishness, that usually indicates that shadow vows are emergent in the relationship.

Hatred

Helping couples become more aware of what were previously unacceptable and often unsavory thoughts, feelings, and emotions helps fully unearth shadow vows. Winnicott's normalizing of countertransference hate in child/caregiver and patient/analyst dyads can be extended to partners locked in relational strife.[35] Hillman notes, "whole love includes hatred as creativity includes destruction."[36]

Normalizing previously unacceptable feelings—even hatred, when the partners have promised to love one another—often reduces the intensity of negative projection and introjection. As each partner recognizes their own feelings, they are less likely to immediately evacuate them out onto another. They can work with the intensity of their feelings, explore them, and track them to their sources which are most often found internally. Relationships then grow more spacious now that there is room enough to hold and work with some hatred as well as love, some anger as well as sweetness.

Abandonment

Shadow vows also reveal themselves when themes of abandonment and betrayal are present. This is evident in the overt infidelities that couples bring to therapy, but there are also other breaches in trust that often undergird the suffering experienced in relationship. Examples of these abandonments include the rejection of sexual advances, choosing family of origin members or friends over a partner, abandoning the relationship to invest fully in the life of a child or children, or choosing creative work or professional career at the expense of the relationship.

Sometimes, an emotional or sexual affair by one partner comes on the heels of the more subtle abandonments of the other partner. Hillman writes, "the broken promise or broken trust is at the same time a breakthrough onto another level of consciousness."[37] If a couple can tolerate the truth of what has happened between them, they may ultimately come to see the betrayal as a symptom of a wounded and wounding relationship that had been crying out for attention long before any thought of straying arose. While unfortunate and painful, the affair may also have been a necessity since they ignored all the other warning signs. Something egregious enough has happened to finally get everyone's attention.

Helping partners voice their shadow vows often leads to the realization that other relationships, albeit less formalized, also come with vows and shadow vows. The issue for someone may not be abandonment *per se* but the challenge of keeping multiple *metaphorical marriages* alive, especially when the obligation to one competes with the obligation to another, as mentioned earlier. For example, how to be mother and wife, or caregiver and working professional when each one demands a sustained commitment of time and energy, or how to manage when urgent situations shuffle their priority? One can quickly become lost amid these multiple commitments, giving new meaning to the tension between the need for intimacy and autonomy.

Selfishness

Union is the dominant archetypal pattern in intimate relationships. During the so-called honeymoon period, couples can easily negotiate issues both large, such as *Where shall we live?* and small, *How much quiet do you need, and when?* Anything less than accommodation might be construed as self-ishness or an inability or unwillingness to give oneself completely to the rela-tionship. Eventually, individual needs begin to resurface. The explorations of shadow vows help couples name the ways their efforts at selflessness have become oppressive. Working with shadow vows serves psychic spaciousness by making room for other archetypal patterns of relating to emerge.

For instance, the desire for solitude may seem like selfishness, but what if it is self-preservation? The necessity of solitude is particularly acute for introverts or for individuals who have learned to be compliant and for whom all human relationship is accommodation. This may be true for couples who attempt to comply with cultural expectations of happiness, especially during the honey-moon period. When partners try to fit their relationship into only one archetypal pattern, union, it can quickly become coercive and suffocating. Then, shadow needs begin to stir. Couples can transform fears about being selfish into a renewed commitment to the archetype of wholeness, the Self.

Conclusion: In Praise of Playfulness

Jung's concept of the shadow is crucial to understanding the fullness of couples' conflicts, particularly those that appear to be nonrational, longstanding, and seemingly intractable. Emotionally committed relationships are always more than they appear to be on the surface. Lurking in the shadows is painful, some-times shameful, material—unvoiced hopes, desires, needs, and expectations. Couples who enter therapy are often rigid with fear or anger; wholly unwilling to open up to their partner and unwilling to face their own shadow.

During the clinical hour, shadow material can reveal itself in the dry, stiff, straight-jacketed way couples present themselves. They embody rigid self-con-trol, the antithesis of openness. In such cases, the partners have lost the capacity to play with one another—the very thing that may have drawn them together. Even though couples come to therapy to *work* on their issues, therapists can use the ability to play together to assess the relationship's health.

Faced with two unhappy people, therapists might think of the couple as a pair of orphaned imaginal children who need to reclaim the fluidity of play-fulness in order to help them satisfy these inner child needs for "mother and father, feeding and protection, omnipotence and idealizations."[38] Play is also characteristic of humanity's most sacred endeavors, including ritual and fes-tival.[39] Winnicott, for whom playing was a given for human life and funda-mentally therapeutic, asserts "only in playing is communication possible."[40]

The invitation to remain playful and cultivate imaginal play space requires ongoing vulnerability, a recurrent theme throughout the chapter. Sadly, the Protestant work ethic, that persistent overlay in America with its counterparts in other cultures, undervalues play within relationships (and life). The Pro-testant work ethic also celebrates heroic invulnerability, self-domination and self-control. It is the antithesis of the attitude needed to invite playfulness and welcome the shadow as teacher. When emotional vulnerability is banished to the shadows, it is impossible for partners to walk the path of individuation alone or together. It becomes impossible for them to support and play with one another in the process of mutual discovery that is one of the great gifts of intimacy.

Notes

1 Portions of this chapter appear in a different form in Nelson & Delmedico 2023.
2 Freud 1960, p. 3.
3 Freud (1933) summarizes the work: "Where the id was, there the ego shall be," and he likened the unconscious to a lake that could be drained in the pursuit of conscious awareness (p. 80). Jung fundamentally departs, believing it to be fathomless.
4 Stein 1998, p. 106.
5 Stein 1998, p. 106.
6 Johnson 1991, pp. 3–4.
7 Johnson 1991, p. 3.
8 Bly 1988, p. 18.
9 Jung 1958, para. 306.
10 Jung 1939, para. 513.
11 Jung 1937, para. 134.
12 Jung 1958, paras 14–18.
13 Jung 1954a, para. 61.
14 Moore 2000, p. v.
15 Reid 2010, n.p.
16 Woodman & Dickson 1996.
17 Jung 1954b, para 179.
18 Bly 1988, p. 18.
19 Jung 1946, para. 503.
20 Wheelwright 1959, p. 58.
21 Nelson, 2012.
22 Jung 1959, para. 123.
23 Moore 1992, p. 30.
24 Moore 1992, p. 30.
25 Bly 1988.
26 Pickering 2008, p. 133.
27 Hollis 2013.
28 Jung 1996, pp. 5–6.
29 Jung 1970, para. 195.
30 See Reich 1973[1945] and Lowen 1971.
31 Whyte 2009.
32 Hillman 1983, p. 187.
33 Jung 1946.
34 Gottman & Gottman 2015.
35 Winnicott 1949.
36 Hillman 1972, p. 88.
37 Hillman 1989a, p. 67.
38 Hillman 1989b, p. 15.
39 Huizinga 2014[1938].
40 Winnicott 1971, p. 73.

References

Bly, R. (1988). *A little book on the human shadow*, W. Booth (ed.). HarperSanFrancisco.
Freud S. (1933). New Introductory Lectures. *SE*. XXII.
Freud S. (1960). *The ego and the id*. W.W. Norton & Co.
Gottman, J. & Gottman, J. (2015). *10 principles for doing effective couples therapy*. New York: W. W. Norton & Co.
Hillman, J. (1972). *The myth of analysis*. Northwestern University Press.
Hillman, J. (1983). *Healing fiction*. Spring Publications.
Hillman, J. (1989a) Betrayal. In *Loose ends* (pp. 63–81). Spring Publications.
Hillman, J. (1989b). Abandoning the child. In *Loose ends* (pp. 5–48). Spring Publications.
Hollis, J. (2013). *Hauntings*. Chiron.
Huizinga, J. (2014). *Homo ludens*. Roy. (Original work published 1938.)
Johnson, R. (1991). *Owning your own shadow*. HarperSanFrancisco.
Jung, C. G. (1937). Psychology and religion. *CW* 11.
Jung, C. G. (1939). Conscious, unconscious, and individuation. *CW* 9i.
Jung, C. G. (1946). The psychology of the transference. *CW* 16.
Jung, C. G. (1954a). Archetypes of the collective unconscious. *CW* 9i.
Jung, C. G. (1954b). Psychological aspects of the mother archetype. *CW* 9i.
Jung, C. G. (1958). Two essays in analytical psychology. *CW* 7
Jung, C. G. (1959). Aion, researches into the phenomenology of the Self. *CW* 9ii.
Jung, C. G. (1970). Civilization in transition. *CW* 10.
Jung, C. G. (1996). *Psychology of kundalini yoga*. Princeton University Press.
Lowen, A. (1971). *The language of the body*. Collier Macmillan.
Moore, T. (1992). *Care of the soul*. HarperCollins.
Moore, T. (2000). *Original self*. HarperCollins.
Nelson, E. (2012). *Psyche's knife*. Chiron.
Nelson, E. E., & Delmedico, A. (2023). When left hands touch: Shadow vows and Jung's quaternity. *Journal of Analytical Psychology*, 68(1), 48–70. https://doi.org/10.1111/1468-5922.12882.
Pickering, J. (2008). *Being in love*. Taylor and Francis.
Reich, W. (1973). *Character analysis* (V. Carfagno, Trans.; 3rd ed.). WRM Press. (Original work published 1945.)
Reid, A. (2010). *Marion Woodman dancing in the flames*. [film]. Capri Vision.
Stein, M. (1998). *Jung's map of the soul*. Open Court.
Van der Kolk, B. (2015). *The body keeps the score*. Viking.
Wheelwright, P. (1959). *Heraclitus*. Oxford University Press.
Whyte, D. (2009). *The three marriages*. Riverhead Books.
Winnicott, D. W. (1949). Hate in the counter-transference. *International Journal of Psycho-analysis*, 30, 69–74.
Winnicott, D. W. (1971). *Playing and reality*. Routledge.
Woodman, M., & Dickson, E. (1996). *Dancing in the flames*. Shambhala.

Chapter 6

The Alchemy of Relationship

Sooner or later, every new understanding about ourselves and one another is subjected to the undercurrents of change. This inevitability may also be the only immutable truth about relationships, as well.[1] One or both partners change. Circumstances change. The relationship itself changes or starts to demand change. The study of alchemy gave Jung a meta-framework for working with these truths. It also provides an excellent lens through which to consider the dynamics that couples bring to therapy.

Jung first encountered alchemy in his early 50s when he read the Taoist alchemical treatise *The Secret of the Golden Flower*.[2] By then, he had already introduced his theories on complexes, typology, archetypes, synchronicity, the collective unconscious, the Self, and individuation. Alchemy provided him with the historical foundations and justification for the whole of his analytical psychology, declaring that one was the "exact equivalent" of the other.[3] His research and writing on alchemy[4] occupied the last 30 years of his life[5] and is an exhaustive exploration into the psychological processes of coming together and coming apart, both within one's self and with others in relationship. With the grounding of his theoretical formulation of transference and countertransference[6] in a sixteenth-century alchemical text, the *Rosarium Philosophorum*,[7] Jung left little doubt that he considered alchemy crucial to understanding relational dynamics.

Some early alchemists were experimenters trying to convert base materials into gold, others searched for an elixir to provide longevity or immortality, while still others were trying to rediscover an "ancient wisdom" lost with the ages.[8] While quick to be dismissed as an antiquated pseudoscience, alchemy is just as alive today with the production of artificial diamonds and our preoccupations with attempts to maintain youthful appearances and extend human life.

The earliest surviving alchemical texts date from the second century and have been found in many different parts of the world, beginning in the Far East, India, and the Middle East. Later manuscripts from the 1200s through the 1800s are found throughout Europe.[9] The texts use heavily symbolic language and cryptic imagery and are difficult to decipher. Whereas historians of science see alchemy as a predecessor of modern chemistry and strip it of all symbolic and mythologic aspects, historians of religion focus on its sacred rites and mystic

DOI: 10.4324/9781032688008-7

symbolism. Jung, on the other hand, approaches alchemy from a *psychological* vantage point.[10] He identifies the alchemists' texts, imagery, and even the work itself as a projection of the unconscious mind into the material world.[11]

The alchemists used all sorts of equipment to carry out their investigations. Through trial and error, they crafted a variety of vessels or *retorts* that could withstand their work's sometimes extreme conditions and pressures. As a result, alchemists often emphasized the importance of proper containment.[12] Similarly, psychologists, each in their own way, have also stressed the containing and holding aspects of the mind, relationships, and therapy.[13] In modern-day consulting rooms (psychological *retorts*), therapists work with the heat and pressure generated by troubled (and troubling) partners. Therapists can thus re-imagine themselves as contemporary alchemists tending the unending processes of change at work in their holding containers. And like the alchemists, today's therapists also project their unconscious material.[14] Schwartz-Salant cautions, "One cannot enter creatively into an interactive field without doing harm unless one is able to accept the often shocking awareness of one's unconscious, shadow qualities which can accompany the process and disrupt one's narcissistic equilibrium."[15] In this case, the projections and countertransferences are onto and into partners, couples, relationships, and even the process of therapy itself.

Each individual psyche is a *retort* holding its own *prima materia* or base material—all the muck and stuff of life.[16] As an alchemical vessel in its own right, the psyche is continually subjected to the full array of ongoing mental processes both conscious and unconscious.[17] By introducing just these two terms, *retort* and *prima materia*, therapists can begin to re-imagine the nature of their work in ways more faithful to the ebbs and flows of actual human experience. Alchemically attuned therapists also actively tend their own *retorts* and *prima materia* as the vicissitudes of therapy demand.

This chapter introduces a few of the provoking, enigmatic, and often psychoactive images from the medieval alchemical corpus. As you encounter the images, let your eyes and mind rest on each one and allow it to penetrate. Notice what emerges as you consider the forces at work in the psyche. What resonates? What gets stirred or illuminated? For example, consider the image in Figure 6.1 taken from a seventeenth-century alchemical manuscript. Think about the conscious and unconscious psychological processes involved in the alchemy of inner work.

As you let your eyes wander and wonder over this image, consider the depth and mystery of your own ongoing inner processes.

Alchemically, when individuals come together, something altogether new is created. Their relationship becomes a third thing—another alchemical vessel or *retort*. Partners tend this *retort* and, in turn, are then subjected to its pressures and demands. Therapists help identify the "stuff" or *prima materia* that is activating for a couple. As co-tenders of these *retorts*, couples therapists can remain curious about the alchemical actions or processes that might be occurring for each of the partners individually and in the relationship itself. At a basic level, alchemically attuned couples therapists observe when things are heating up, cooling down, dissolving, or

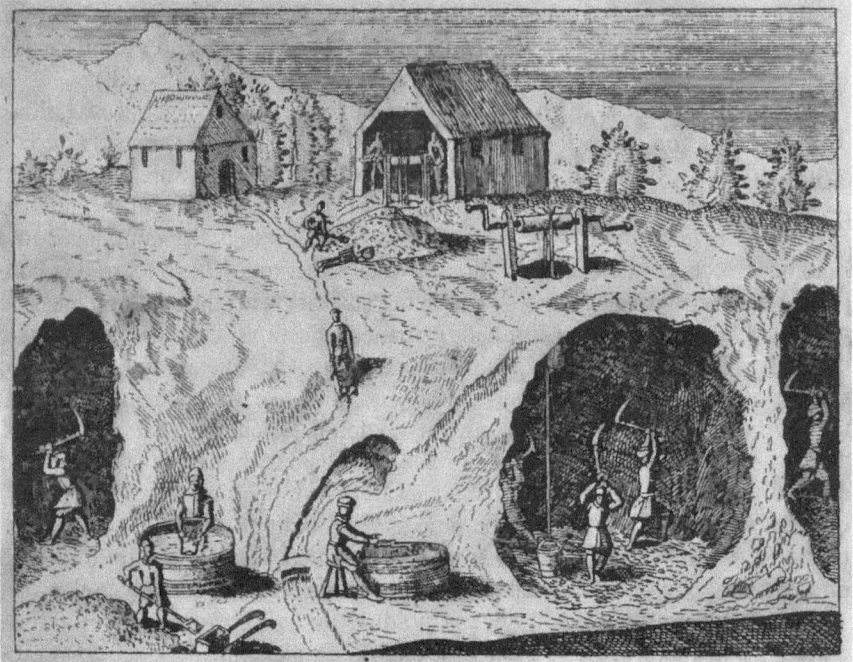

Figure 6.1 Of Fossilized Earth. Reprinted from *Septimana Philosophica* (p. 67), by M. Maier, 1620. Jennis. Public domain. Courtesy of the Getty Research Institute.

coming together for each partner and the relationship. Sensing even subtle changes, therapists can ask, *What is happening right now between you two?*

Next, consider the image in Figure 6.2. Imagine yourself as the therapeutic alchemist on one knee tending the flame and heat of the *retort* or alchemical bath. A man with a dove on his head is shown in the waters, but one can easily reimagine the bath to be holding a couple alchemically steeped and stewing in the *prima materia* of their relationship.

Continue to focus on Figure 6.2, but now imagine *yourself* as the figure in the alchemical bath. As it is for therapists in daily practice today, the alchemists of old did the work, and the work also worked on them. Whether therapists know it or not (or want to admit it), they are also stewing in the work, hour over clinical hour. And sometimes, the stewing continues long after. Often, the mind is far from finished with sessions at the end of a clinical hour or day. To realize this alchemical effect, clinicians need only to notice thoughts and moods continuing of their own accord long after sessions have ended.

Alchemy does not replace current therapeutic practice or clinical training. Rather, it transforms the framework and enlarges the therapist's holding capacity when they are confronted with the mysteries inherent in every relationship. Couples therapists strive daily to help transform base material (i.e., the "shit" of

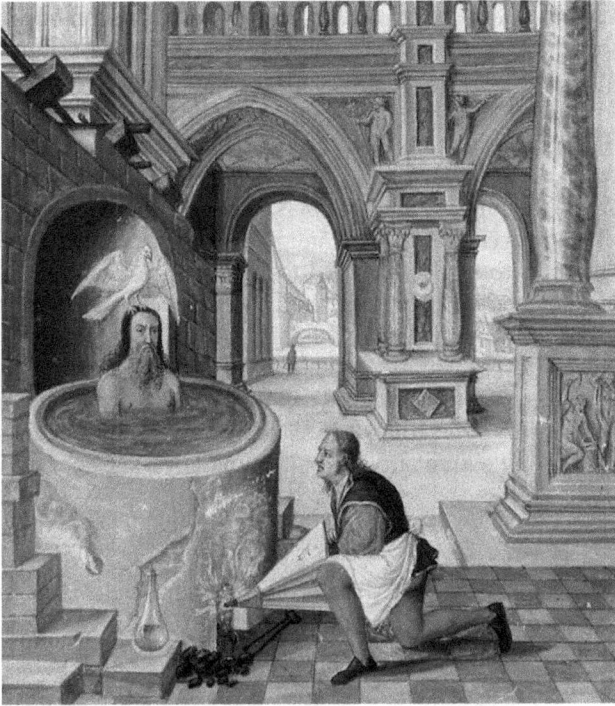

Figure 6.2 The Alchemical Bath (Plate XI). Reprinted from *Splendor Solis*, by S. Trismosin, 1582. Kegan Paul, Trench, Trübner & Co. Public domain.

the partners' lives) into gold. And it is not just ordinary gold (*aurum vulgi*), but the same philosophical gold that the alchemists were seeking.[18]

Alchemical Processes

Throughout the centuries, alchemists used imagery and writing to codify, often with contradiction and vagueness, the many different procedures, directions, and stages required to produce their desired ends.[19] They conceptualized their work in a multitude of ways. Jung noted the intrapsychic and relational dynamics of the alchemists' accounts and, through careful study of medieval European alchemical texts, elaborated the psychological meaning of the processes.[20]

Reimagining the consulting rooms as *retorts* filled with couples' *prima materia* should not constitute much of a leap for marriage and family therapists for one reason: another word alchemists used for *retort* was *crucible*, a term David Schnarch adopts in his formulation of the sexual and marital container for couples[21] and which Napier and Whitaker use to capture the felt sense of the intense forces encountered when working with families.[22] Things get hot (or cold) fast in consulting rooms when partners begin to air old wounds. The alchemy of tears can flood containers, but they can also sometimes dissolve long-held grievances. Therapists tend these unceasing alchemical processes as their action plays out in the lives of partners and their relationships.

The skill of *tending* the retort or crucible of the relationship recalls the roots of the word psychotherapy. From the original Greek, therapy, or *therapeuein*, meant "to tend" or "to listen," and psyche meant soul.[23] James Hollis,[24] Lionel Corbett,[25] James Hillman,[26] and Thomas Moore,[27] among others, remind us that psychotherapy is care of the soul in anguish. Rather than reducing couples and their symptoms to things that need fixing, curing, or saving, an alchemical perspective invites therapists to tend the processes at work in couples' *retorts* which are ever-transformative. As such, the idea of progress, especially *linear* progress, may not accord with the meandering ways of the soul in relationship.

The alchemical processes described below can help therapists organize the chaos or *massa confusa* that couples bring to therapy. They can also be used to help track the shifting nature of couples' dynamics over the course of treatment.

Calcinatio

Calcinatio, the Latin term for calcination, is a fiery alchemical process that uses high heat to drive off impurities and reduce substances to purer forms.[28] See the medieval depiction of *calcinatio* in Figure 6.3.[29]

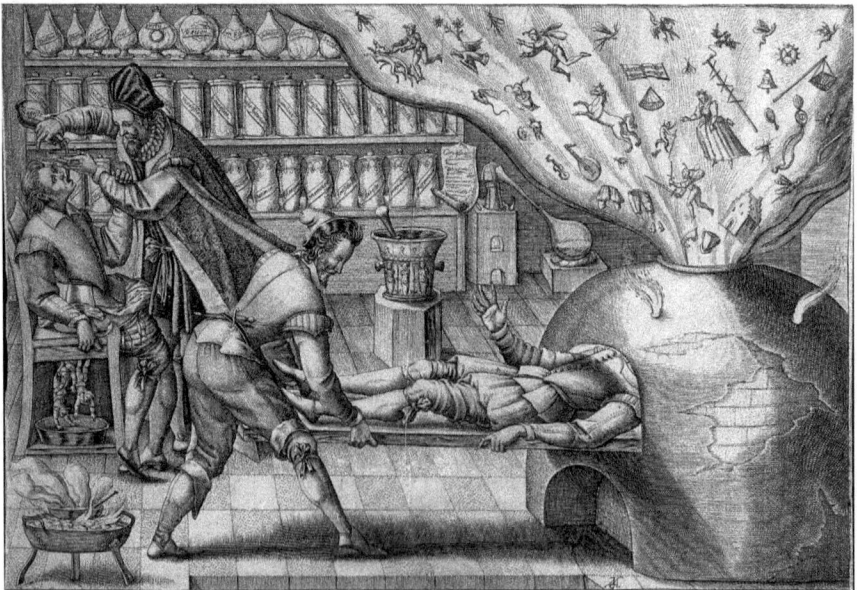

Figure 6.3 Mathieu Greuter. (c. 1600). *A Surgery Where All Fantasy and Follies Are Purged and Good Qualities Are Prescribed.* [line engraving]. Wellcome Collection. Public domain.

An alchemically attuned therapist can observe *calcinatio* occurring when, after much struggle and toil in therapy (psychic heat), there comes a reduction of confusion, and a couple begins to have more clarity about their situation.[30] The sheer dint of therapeutic action can drive off fog surrounding past circumstances or events and produce new insight. Instead of participating in meandering, hazy sessions, couples are now able to express essential realizations and concisely summarized truths. It is challenging for therapists to tend the high heat of *calcinatio* in a couple's *retort* when partners argue, bicker, and fight. But their heated efforts can serve to drive off misperceptions and distortions in the relationship and produce something potentially more authentic for themselves.

Calcinatio is but one process in the alchemy of couples therapy. As many therapists know, gaining some clarity is only a preliminary stage in the work. For example, when betrayals come to light, or there is a loss, a couple is now faced with what to do with this purer truth, this alchemical salt. Jung offers a distinction between suffering and wisdom that has alchemical implications: "Tears, sorrow, and disappointment are bitter, but wisdom is the comforter in all psychic suffering ... where there is bitterness wisdom is lacking, and where wisdom is there can be no bitterness."[31] It can take considerable, grueling alchemical clinical work for couples to transform bitterness into new wisdom.

Calcinatio occurs at other moments in couples therapy, for instance when either or both partners complain that they are being driven crazy by the other or when a therapist finds themselves expressing attitudes or reacting in ways that overtly frustrate a couple. These all add heat to the clinical material, sometimes consciously but often unconsciously. *Calcinatio* is also at work whenever partners share secrets, releasing the residue of bound-up shame, guilt, anxiety, or fear.[32] The fires of *calcinatio* sometimes burn most intensely in the sexual frustrations and unrequited desires that often go unspoken in couples therapy. (Couples tend to bury them under their "communication problems.") Fully tending the process of *calcinatio* helps unearth these deeper and purer truths which a couple previously could not have realized or held.

Solutio

Solutio is the watery alchemical process of dissolving.[33] It works differently at various stages of relationship. *Solutio* occurs when therapists help couples dissolve solidified long-held beliefs that may have been causing them so much trouble. *Solutio* can also happen when there is a "loosening of a cramped attitude"[34] or when a partner's hardened heart dissolves.[35] See the alchemical *solutio* shown in Figure 6.4. Since couples are rarely proactive in seeking therapy, this image characterizes the state of many relationships by the time partners arrive for therapy.

Alchemically, the couple intimates, *The King (our relationship) is in trouble. We have done all we know to do to save it. We have used all of our royal powers to no avail. We are here with no small measure of desperation and exasperation and some real doubts as to the possibility of rescue.*

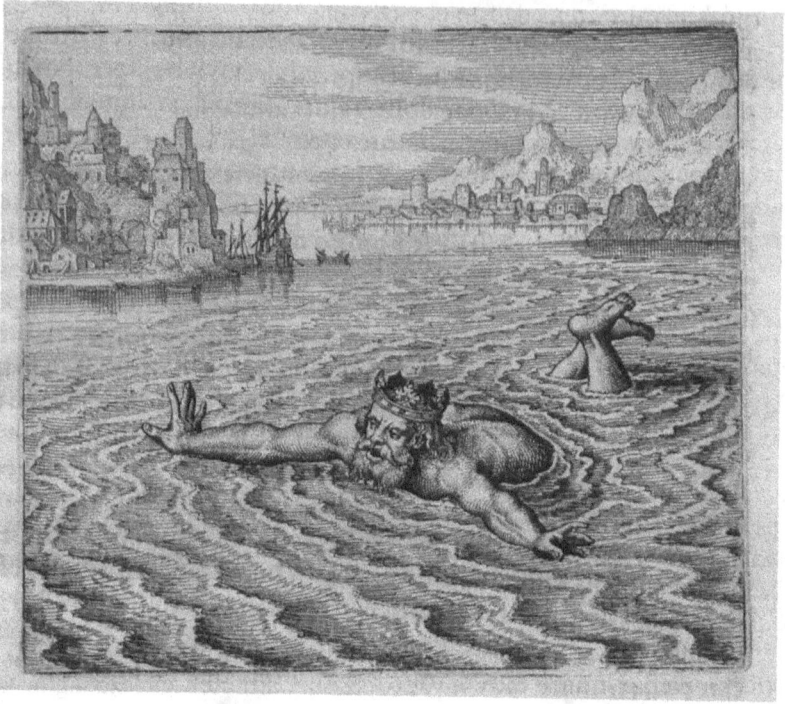

Figure 6.4 The King Swimming in the Sea, Crying With a Loud Voice (Emblem XXXI). Reprinted from *Atalanta Fugiens* (p. 133), by M. Maier, 1618. Johann-Theodor de Bry. Public domain. Courtesy of Science History Institute.

Some couples experience an altogether different kind of *solutio* when one partner acts as a psychological container for the dissolving other.[36] Their (often unconscious) agreement is: *You can dissolve into me, and I will hold you and us.* As one partner regresses, under-functions, and under-develops, the other finds purpose in holding and over-functioning. Over time, couples can become archetypally entrenched in these roles, making change exceedingly difficult.

When partners opt for premarital counseling, therapists witness another kind of *solutio*. At this enchanting stage of relationship, deep connection and heightened passions are the order of the day. Both partners have largely lost their ego boundaries and their separateness and have dissolved into one another. They are now more couple than individual and have gone unconscious together into a blissful state.[37] With differences vanishing and harmony reigning supreme, thoughts of not only being together, but being together *forever* naturally arise. How else but at the mercy of *solutio* do our fairy tales of happily-ever-after arise?

Couples therapists are sometimes called upon to help tend an altogether different *solutio*: the dissolving of a relationship. This type of *solutio* has been at work long before some couples arrive in therapy; their relationship is already all but over. In these instances, alchemical work with couples helps both partners more fully realize what they may have already known on unconscious levels.

Coagulatio

Coagulatio, or coagulation, is an earthy alchemical intermediate process where things become solidified.[38] Psychologically, *coagulatio* occurs when things come into focus and find some stability in the conscious mind. Creativity and ego development are also associated with *coagulatio*. Trauma-trained EMDR[39] therapists will notice *coagulatio* during reprocessing when a new cognition emerges in the patient's mind. For example, a patient's long-held belief that they should have put up more of a fight during abuse suddenly forms into the realization that they were just a child without the possibility of agency.

Coagulatio occurs with couples when aspects of each partner's individual identity gains substance and when new ideas about their relationship or ways of being with one another coalesce. From an alchemical perspective, their identity as a couple forms and re-forms in an ever-emergent process. In the aftermath of *coagulatio*, partners can struggle if they hold too tightly to newly conceived ideas about themselves, each other, or the relationship. Sooner or later, other alchemical processes (always at work in relationships) begin transforming these new hard-won perspectives.

Couples who complain about being stuck experience a different asspect of *coagulatio*. Therapists recognize this *coagulatio* when couples repeatedly share the same litany of grievances without gaining any new insight.[40] Therapists can call attention to the repetitive nature of the complaints, noting the sense of stuckness for a couple rather than trying to fight it. For example, therapists can say, *It feels like you are both stuck here again, at this same place. Does it feel that way to you? If so, how?* They can inquire further, asking, *As we talk about it today, though it feels the same, what do you notice that is different about it?* Helping couples locate themselves in their stuckness gives them an expanded language and framework to hold themselves during this stage.

Coagulatio is also at work when partners complain of being weighed down or held back. See the alchemical representation of *coagulatio* in Figure 6.5 depicting an eagle chained to a toad.

More broadly, the work of therapy itself can be re-visioned using one of alchemy's oldest axioms, *Solve et coagula* (dissolve and coagulate).[41] Ideas, beliefs, feelings, traumas, anxieties, depressions, joys, insights, failures—all of the psychic material brought to couples therapy—are repeatedly worked and reworked, dissolved, and coagulated in this great alchemical endeavor until they can rest easier in the soul and the relationship. Therapists and couples also know they are experiencing *coagulatio* when the heat and energy around the things they have been wrestling with have dissipated.

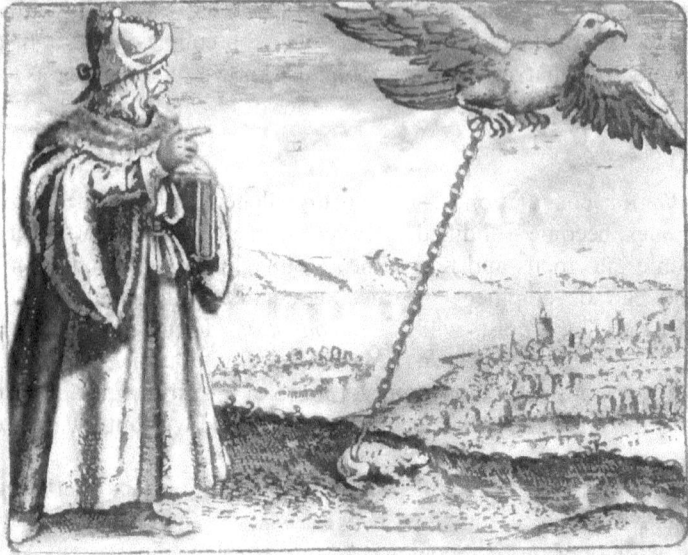

Figure 6.5 Eagle and Toad. Reprinted from *Symbola Aureae Mensae Duodecim Nationum* (p. 192), by M. Maier, 1617. Antonij Hummij. Public domain. Courtesy of the National Central Library of Rome.

Mortificatio

Mortificatio, also known as *putrefactio* or *nigredo*, is the alchemical process of decay, dying, deadness, rotting, and composting.[42] *Mortificatio* places unique demands on the psyche, making it a challenging process for couples therapists to faithfully attend. *Mortificatio* is at work when therapists have a sense that no matter what a couple (or therapist) tries, things only get worse. There can be an overwhelming sense of stagnation and deadness. Couples and therapists experience impatience and despair during this seemingly fallow and fruitless period as a necessary contraction is taking place.

In couples therapy, *mortificatio* may occur when there is a loss of hope with no sign of progress or change.[43] The stagnation of *mortificatio* makes it hard to remember that active processes—dying, rotting, and composting—are still working out of sight in the depths of the relationship. *Mortificatio* is reminiscent of St. John of the Cross's dark night of the soul.[44] Alchemists describe this period of darkness as a "black blacker than black."[45] Therapists are not usually trained to attend the extended periods of darkness that is *mortificatio*. Instead, we must look to the writers and philosophers, the other experts in the alchemy of human suffering. One of author Toni Morrison's characters instructs us on the proper therapeutic orientation when working in *mortificatio*.

And talking about dark! You think dark is just one color, but it ain't. There're five or six kinds of black. Some silky, some woolly. Some just empty. Some like fingers. And it don't stay still. It moves and changes from one kind of black to another. Saying something is pitch black is like saying something is green. What kind of green? Green like my bottles? Green like a grasshopper? Green like a cucumber, lettuce, or green like the sky is just before it breaks loose to storm? Well, night black is the same way. May as well be a rainbow.[46]

Chinese philosopher Lao-Tzu encourages us to see the "darkness within darkness" because it is "the gateway to all understanding."[47] Confronted with so much darkness day in and day out, it becomes difficult for therapists working under the influence of the wounded healer archetype[48] to stay down in it long enough for their therapeutic eyes to adjust. Additionally, textbooks, coursework, and trainings tend to focus on theory and technique as applied to vignettes to assist with case conceptualizations, treatment plans, and interventions, all in service of moving patients and couples "up" and "out" of their psychological discomforts, as opposed to "down" and "in" and "through" them.

Getting comfortable with *mortificatio* is useful because it accounts for the soul's natural movement downward and inward toward death, an essential yet neglected phase of psychic and coupled life.[49] The heroic ego wants immediate relief, yet the relentless pursuit of improvement induces its own form of unique suffering. Unfortunately, one cannot move from one psychological truth to another without the painful destruction of the former. Any psychological (or spiritual) change involves *mortification* as old ideas and beliefs that worked so well for so long begin to decay of their own accord.

Hillman attributes this tendency for decay to the natural pathologizing function of the psyche that serves to temper the soul.[50] For example, in relationships, the old ways of loving and being together simply begin to not work anymore. Unfortunately, the mind cannot easily let go because new ways of being together have not yet emerged. A full tending of *mortificatio* is required for old ways to die off in order to open up space, a pregnant space, between partners for new ways of connecting (or disconnecting) to emerge.

Mortificatio is miserable for everyone, including the therapist. All attempts to relieve a couple's suffering are in vain during this stage. *Mortificatio*, that most natural of alchemical processes, does not ask for alleviation. Rather it asks for gentle facilitation of the suffering inherent in the decay, dying, death, and composting processes needed to fertilize the emergent psychic life of a couple and their relationship. So, alchemically speaking, therapists are not agents of improvement but tenders of *mortificatio*, the dying process. In this case, it is the death of anything that no longer fits for a couple: outgrown ideas, beliefs, philosophies, and ways of being together. See the couple's *mortificatio* portrayed in the alchemical image in Figure 6.6. Also, notice the figures tending the process.

Through an alchemical lens, couples' issues are no longer perceived as problems to be dealt with or obstacles to be overcome. Instead, they can be viewed as things

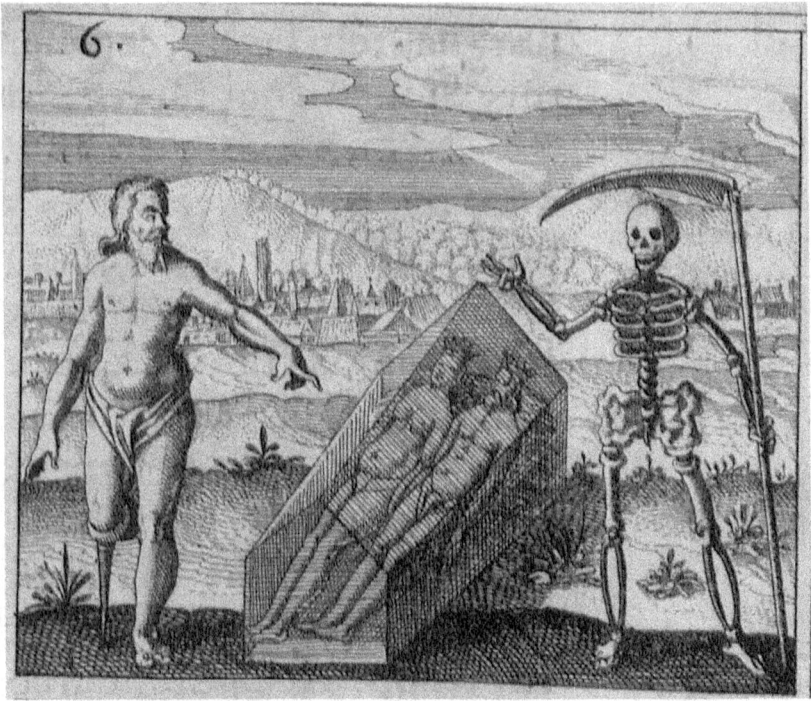

Figure 6.6 Mortificatio. Reprinted from *Philosophia Reformata* (p. 243), by Johann Mylius, 1622. Jennis. Public domain. Courtesy of the Foundation of the Works of C. G. Jung, Zurich.

that may need to die. The work is to see if a couple can allow the things that no longer serve them to decay, die, and rot away. An alchemically attuned therapist tends this process while also tending the fears about the unknown future ahead as well as the grief, sadness, and anger over the dying things or things long since dead.

After working through the darkness of *mortificatio*, a couple's wellspring of resilience, creativity, and (re)generativity naturally becomes available. Coming together again in a more authentic way—if it is a couple's fate to do so—is a process that usually takes care of itself without the need for a therapist and their prescriptions of date nights and getaways because an altogether new flame, alchemically purified, now burns in the couple's hearts.

Separatio

Separatio, the alchemical process of separation is fundamental to any therapeutic endeavor.[51] It is perhaps the predominant process at play in therapy. By the time couples arrive in treatment, many are suffering under the alchemical action of *separatio*. The blissful feeling of being dissolved together during *solutio* is now a distant memory. Partners are no longer completing each other's thoughts and sentences and embers from the fires of passion have grown cold. Couples must sort out and re-imagine themselves again as individuals, only this time as individuals in a committed relationship.

Separatio occurs in a variety of other ways in couples therapy. It can be a monumental task to separate partners from their problems long enough for them to have some other vantage point to evaluate their difficulties. Projections of problems onto (or into) partners can be difficult to separate out and withdraw. The previous wounding couples bring into a relationship and project onto their partner must also be clarified and worked through. Jung reminds us that there are always "hooks" for these projections that tend to be "sticky;" removing them is no small task.[52] When one partner has become the identified patient, which sometimes happens in family systems, the alchemical action of *separatio* can help distinguish the person from the problem.

See the image in Figure 6.7, and reflect on the tremendous and often messy effort required in assisting couples with sorting their psychological material.

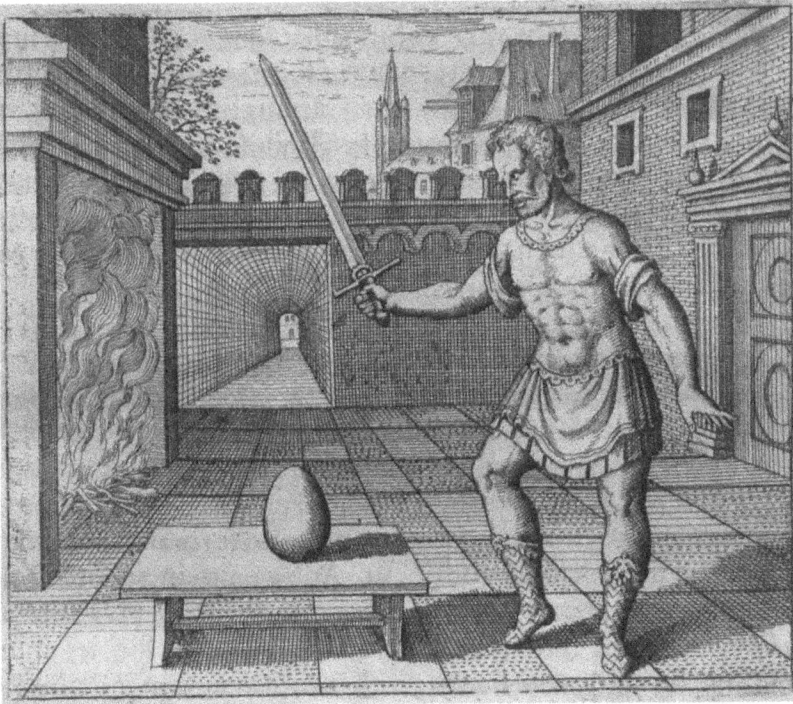

Figure 6.7 On the Secrets of Nature. Take the Egg and Strike It With the Fiery Sword (Emblem VIII). Reprinted from *Atalanta Fugiens* (p. 41), by M. Maier, 1618. Johann-Theodor de Bry. Public domain. Courtesy of Science History Institute.

Ibn Sina, the tenth-century Islamic philosopher and alchemist, emphasizes the importance of *separatio*: "Purify husband and wife separately, so that they may unite more intimately; for if you do not purify them, they cannot love each other."[53] Relationships are healthiest when partners can be "alone together," deeply connected, yet distinctly individual.[54] Yet couples fear the process of *separatio* because it comes with the loss of powerfully positive projections as the relationship tries to ground itself in reality for the first time. The spell is breaking as the clock strikes midnight, the princess is trading the gown for cinder-smudged rags, and the prince is turning back into a frog. In this time of *separatio*, couples bring all their ashes and warts to therapy, arriving panicky and confused.

Separatio is also required for partners to fully mature and leave their families of origin. A more complete separation from parents is often necessary to authentically engage with one's partner. This process is also painful for parents who have not done their own psychological work. Considering the secrets that individuals and couples keep from parents and their reluctance to share preferences and their authentic selves, this is no small developmental achievement. *Separatio* is at work in the individuation process as couples psychologically mature and differentiate.

The painful sorting of the commingled sludge at the heart of a relationship (or bottom of the *retort*) also requires *separatio*. This sludge contains the couple's individual and interlocked complexes, which form battle lines for relational conflict (see Chapter 2). The ongoing work of *separatio* distinguishes what belongs to whom in a relationship, and it aids in the withdrawal of projections.[55]

Separatio can also be seen in the breaking up or divorce stage of relationships and includes physical, material, psychological, and spiritual separations, each occurring in varying degrees and on their own timetable. Thomas Moore's excellent treatment of endings in *Soul Mates* reminds the heroic fantasy-suffused ego that, ultimately, no one escapes *separatio* as all things, ourselves included, are subject to the natural cycle of beginnings, middles, and endings.[56]

The last great *separatio* is death itself. If a partner is not able to separate themselves enough from a departed loved one, sometimes another death quickly follows. Alchemically attuned therapists are sometimes called upon to tend this heart-wrenching and most painful work with couples when either or both partners are faced with impermanence.

Coniunctio

Coniunctio, or union, is the great goal or *opus* of the alchemical endeavor. It is also the goal for couples wishing to reconnect and stay together. *Coniunctio* is often symbolized in alchemical imagery by marriage or intercourse, or by the union of pairs of opposites including the sun and moon, man and woman, king and queen, brother and sister, human with God, and with the symbol of the hermaphrodite.[57]

It is not a question of whether *two become one* in a sacred union, even though *coniunctio* is sometimes symbolized in wedding ceremonies when partners light a unity candle together and extinguish their individual candles. They certainly do unite—but only while the process of *solutio* is at work in the relationship and they live within that fully dissolved, blissful, Edenlike honeymoon stage. Sooner or later the dissolved, *one-ish* state of togetherness naturally begins to separate and a couple becomes more *two-ish* again. Therapists are called upon to help sort out, hold, and assist couples in tending these growing pains. They can normalize these soulful movements by helping couples recognize their first big *coniunctio* as an authentic coming together and then reframe it as a stage, just one of many stages of relationship.

The alchemical work of *coniunctio* is also needed when couples enter therapy already far removed from one another. They are not in need of reconnecting but of *re-imagining* themselves anew. If a couple attempts to extinguish the candles of individuality this time, trying to dissolve (*solutio*) together again, their effort will not last. Unfortunately, well-meaning therapists, in an effort to encourage a return to the original *solutio*, ask couples how they fell in love and what they first liked about each other. Even if such prompts appear to succeed, the result will be a *lesser coniunctio* that does not hold up for couples at this stage in their relationship. Couples are often painfully aware of previous failed attempts to dissolve together again, but they may make further attempts under a therapist's care. When those attempts inevitably fail too, they are usually no longer willing to continue this painful cycle of hope and despair.

Rather than trying to light a unity candle that will no longer stay lit, therapists can assist couples with a more sustainable *coniunctio*. The partners come together again but, instead of dissolving into one, now the two become three. They remain committed to the relationship while retaining a greater sense of selfhood and separateness as individuals.

While many images of *coniunctio* depict a pair of opposites in some form of union, the alchemical image in Figure 6.8 expresses the notion of separate connectedness and the creation of a third.

Most couples have little trouble surrendering to the mysterious alchemy of falling in love. Many yearn for it, anticipate it, and delight in it. But when the ground underneath the relationship begins to undulate, the heroic ego struggles to prevent fractures in the unity by trying to return to *the way we were* rather than opening to what is actually happening. Any change can be frightening; the ego likes stability, sometimes demanding blissful *solutio* and only *solutio*. But change is inevitable because the two partners have created a third, the relationship, which is a living thing with its own fate. The more couples resist this natural fact, the more they suffer.

Despite the alchemists' efforts, they never achieved the *greater coniunctio* of creating gold, eternal youth, or immortality. They combined many elements into new substances but realized they had achieved only a *lesser coniunctio* each time.

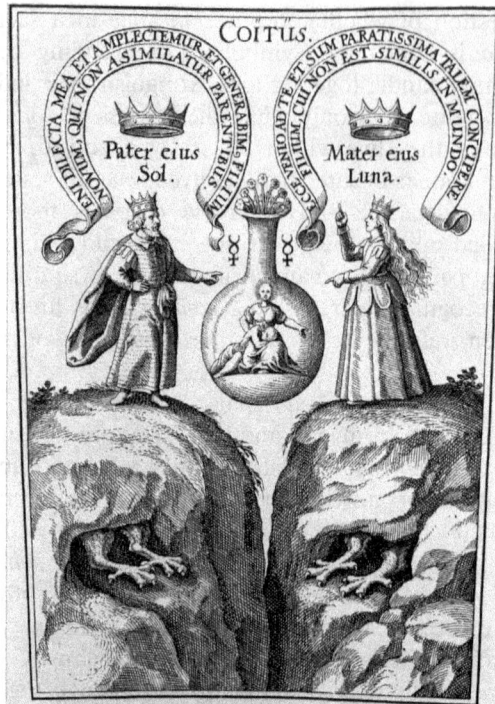

Figure 6.8 Coitus. Reprinted from *Anotomia Auri, Part V* (p. 6), by Johann Mylius, 1628. Jennis. Public domain.

Regardless, the alchemists did not give up the work. They devoted themselves entirely to tending these processes, which ultimately produced their own *alchemical* gold, which they called *the wisdom of the philosophers*. In the processes of psychological alchemy with couples it might be called *the wisdom of the therapists*. Just as any alchemical gold is a *lesser coniunctio* which, sooner or later, must go back into the fires or be dissolved, subjected again to the full array of alchemical processes, so too, any solid place in a relationship must also be melted down or dissolved again (and again) as psyches grow and change.

Alchemically attuned therapists help couples transform their view of relationships from static and binding to alive and ever-emerging—just as the partners are alive and emerging. Relationships, like people, have their own fate. While couples place many explicit and implicit demands on relationships, relationships also place demands on the partners and powerfully influence their individuation. Living relationships that are imagined, re-imagined, and lived anew each day possess a distinctive vitality. They are forever being alchemically reconstituted, one *lesser coniunctio* after another, over a lifetime. This ongoing process of destruction and renewal is symbolized alchemically with the ouroboros (Figure 6.9), the serpent forever devouring its own tail.

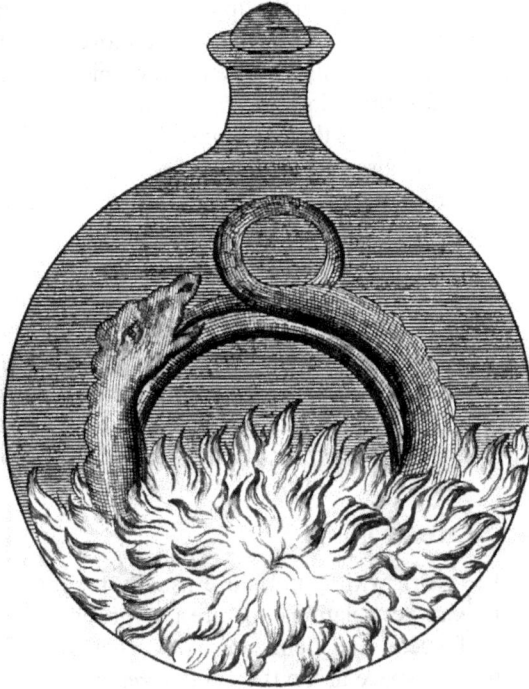

Figure 6.9 Ouroboros. Reprinted from *Elementa Chemiae* (p. 512), by J. C. Barchusen, 1718. Theodorum Haak. Public domain. Courtesy of the Getty Research Institute.

Like the ouroboros, relationships forever devour themselves in the process of renewal. Couples therapists might imagine their work as tending four interconnected flasks, each with its own heat and ouroboros: one for each partner, one for the relationship itself, and one for the therapist who is also called upon to tend their own ongoing process as well.

Alchemy and the Process of Couples Therapy

Another important way that alchemists organized their work was through the use of colored stages, three of the prominent ones being *nigredo* (blackening), *albedo* (whitening), and *rubedo* (reddening). These colored stages also provide a contemporary parallel with the psychological work done with individuals and couples. To track clinical action with couples over the course of treatment, therapists, like alchemists, can imagine the work as beginning in *nigredo*, a state of darkness, blackness, confusion, and despair that couples typically bring into therapy at the outset. Therapists then amplify (*amplificatio*) all manner of clinical material (*prima materia*) in an attempt to make sense of the psychic darkness.

As the work proceeds, and a couple obtains new insights and some relief, an *albedo* or whitening occurs. *Albedo* marks the movement out of darkness and confusion. An overly optimistic couple (or therapist) might believe that a new day has dawned for the relationship, but *albedo* is only a temporary stage. Couples have yet to see if their new insights can stand the test of time. In a way, the *albedo* is a false dawn and not the actual light. A third stage, *rubedo*, uses the fires of blood, sweat, and tears of a daily life lived together to redden or temper these new insights.

Of course, much to the frustration of all egos involved, there is no final goal. (Decentralizing and tempering the ego is an ongoing Herculean task in its own right.) Therapists, like the alchemists, come to realize that the work is circular in nature. This process of *circulatio* brings couples again and again through the stages of *nigredo, albedo* and *rubedo*. Therapists can track a couple's stages with them, helping partners become more comfortable with the ever-changing quality of their relational opus as one intermediate stage segues into another.

An Alchemical State of Mind

Therapists trained to work with couples are usually taught that the relationship is the patient. And yet relationships are comprised of individuals, each with a unique set of needs and demands. An alchemical lens expands the therapist's ability to hold space in the therapeutic *retort* to tend the alchemical processes affecting all three, both partners and the relationship. Over-simplified clinical vignettes used in training cannot make space for the mysteries inherent in the messiness of *actual* relationships. Some therapists insulate themselves from this *massa confusa* by invoking a teacher/student constellation offering worksheets and homework assignments while the subtle and sometimes tectonic alchemical forces at work in relationships are left unacknowledged and untended. In addition to holding what Tavistock's Mary Morgan calls a "couple state of mind,"[58] therapists can also cultivate an alchemical state of mind.

Many therapists seem only to have the stomach for one alchemical process, *coniunctio*, with its promise of reunion and passionate reconnection. Since couples come to treatment under all manner of duress, familiarity with the other alchemical processes can help therapists and the partners hold and more deeply engage painful material. Even though every ego in the room would like a timetable for repair as well as a guarantee, the alchemically informed couples therapist knows that the undulations of the soul of a relationship follow their own rhythm. Couples must live through them to be more authentically connected.

Regardless of which alchemical process or stage is occurring, working through it is never fast, easy, or promising for anyone. It often constellates confusion, despair, frustration, and anger. But tending these unrelenting processes makes it possible for couples to re-imagine themselves and their relationship in the fullness of time, and like any art, it cannot be rushed. Many therapists are taught to hold a position of hope, but the only authentic hope available during extended periods of hopelessness may be an alchemical one. Instead of trying to immediately mitigate a couple's suffering, therapists accept and amplify problems to urge alchemical processes along.[59] If a couple is already cooking in it, then it is important to help them tend the fire and aim for a full and proper cooking rather than trying to douse flames and retard the processes already at work in the soul of the relationship. If they are coming apart, help them examine the specific ways in which they are coming apart.

Never underestimate the power of a couple's problems, for in the wounds lie the alchemical medicine. Therapists can stay *down and in* those wounds with couples by keeping their focus granular. For example, when couples report fighting with one another, therapists can use *separatio* to sort the details of the conflict, the moment-by-moment interactions and recollections. This includes asking a host of specific questions such as, *What did you do and why? What did you really feel like doing instead? Why didn't you do it? What did you say? What did you really want to say, but didn't? Why did you not say it? Were each of you aware of these unspoken choices and feelings? What was going on for each of you psychologically and physically, while all that was going on?* Therapists can also get curious about the partners' present-moment awareness and their individual recollections of other conflicts, by asking, *What is going on now as we revisit it? Does this fight feel familiar, somehow? Where and when have you had these kinds of fights before? With other partners? In your family growing up? What happened in those fights, and what happened afterward?* These *separatio* questions help each partner sort out what was happening for them during the fight as well as connect it to past conflicts. Once they realize how deep, old, and intractable such conflicts are, greater empathy for each other's suffering can occur.

Typically, therapists tend to only listen long enough to identify patterns, then quickly get to work trying to ease couples' tensions and also protect themselves from toxic content. Alchemically attuned therapists are doing something altogether different: they are expertly, faithfully tending a couple's *retort*—simply for its own sake, alert to the alchemical process(es) already at work. For example, when couples are fighting in the full heat of *calcinatio*, alchemical therapists do not quell the argument. Instead, they tend the flames of a couple's discord and teach them to fight fairly. Alchemically productive fighting fosters a fuller working through of the conflict without being destructive to either partner. There are no winners or losers, and no one is right or wrong. No one gets the upper hand, and no one is dominated. There is no violence occurring when couples fight fair. The Gottmans' four horses (criticism, contempt, defensiveness, and stonewalling) are nowhere to be found in productive fighting.[60] There is only some relief and some increased clarity once a hard, painful issue is sorted out. The partners who work through their sludge (*massa confusa*), come away with better understandings of each other and their relationship.

Conclusion

The alchemical processes described in this chapter correlate with the therapist's *felt sense* of the ever-changing dynamics between couples in relationship. Working from an alchemical perspective, therapists can craft a more robust therapeutic container for couples and increase their own capacity to hold a broader range of affect for longer periods. For example, consider the different clinical stances required for working with the blissful *solutio* of new relationships, laboring through an extended period of *mortificatio*, or the painstaking effort demanded of *separatio*. Hillman reminds us that surviving "the fruitlessly bitter and dry periods, the melancholies that never seem to end, the wounds that do not heal, the grinding sadistic mortifications of shame and the putrefactions of love and friendship" are indeed accomplishments, adding that "these are beginnings because they are endings, dissolutions, deconstructions."[61] An alchemical frame of mind accommodates and normalizes a fuller range of material emerging from real relationships over the long arc of coupled life.

This chapter introduced alchemy and some of its terminology. You have been invited to think like an alchemist, talk like an alchemist, imagine like an alchemist, and work like an alchemist. Your work as an alchemically attuned therapist is a *magnum opus* of soul-making, for each partner, for their relationship, and for you.

Notes

1 Schwarz-Salant 1998.
2 Bair 2003.
3 Bair 2003, p. 398.
4 Jung 1944, 1963, 1967.
5 Hanna 1976.
6 Jung 1946.
7 Toltetanus 1550[c. 1200s].
8 Eliade 1971[1956], p. 110.
9 Maxwell-Stuart 2008.
10 Jung 1989[1961].
11 Jung 1944.
12 Fordham 1985.
13 cf. Bion 1962, Winnicott 1972, Jung 1925.
14 Jung 1946.
15 Schwartz-Salant 1998, p. 168.
16 Edinger 1985.
17 Jung 1944.
18 Jung 1944.
19 See Abraham 1998, Aromatico 2000, de Rola 1988, Fabricius 1976, and Roob 2021.
20 Jung 1944.
21 Schnarch 1991.
22 Napier & Whitaker 1978.
23 Hollis 2022, p. 93.

24 Hollis 2022.
25 Corbett 2015.
26 Hillman 1975.
27 Moore 1994.
28 Marlan 2005.
29 While the eye is immediately drawn to the alchemical action of *calcinatio* occurring in the foreground, there are also two figures in the back left. The one standing is pouring liquid from a flask labeled "Wisdom" down the throat of the seated person who is also expelling small court jesters or fools out into a bed pan below the chair.
30 Hillman 2014.
31 Jung 1963, para. 330.
32 Edinger 1985.
33 Edinger 1985.
34 Grinnell 1973, p. 92.
35 Jung 1963, para. 364.
36 Jung 1925.
37 Edinger 1985.
38 Edinger 1985.
39 Eye Movement Desensitization and Reprocessing
40 von Franz 1980.
41 Abraham 1998, p. 186.
42 Marlan 2005.
43 Schwartz-Salant 1998.
44 St. John 1953[1619].
45 Jung 1944, para. 343.
46 Morrison 1977, pp. 40–41.
47 Tzu 1988[c. 400 BCE], p. 1.
48 von Franz 1990.
49 Schwartz-Salant 1998.
50 Hillman 1975.
51 Edinger 1985.
52 Jung 1948, para. 519.
53 Kelly 1893[1676], p. 35.
54 Fisher 2019.
55 Jung 1963
56 Moore 1994.
57 Edinger 1985.
58 Morgan 2019.
59 Jung 1944.
60 Gottman & Gottman 2015.
61 Hillman 2014, pp. 89–90.

References

Abraham, L. (1998). *A dictionary of alchemical imagery.* Cambridge University Press.
Aromatico, A. (2000). *Alchemy* (J. Hawkes, Trans.). Abrams.
Barchusen, J. C. (1718). *Elementa chemiae.* Theodorum Haak. https://archive.org/details/johannisconradib00barc/page/n569/mode/2up.
Bair, D. (2003). *Jung: A biography.* Back Bay Books.
Bion, W. R. (1962). *Learning from experience.* Karnac.

Corbett, L. (2015). *The soul in anguish*. Chiron Publications.

de Rola, S. K. (1988). *The golden game*. Thames Hudson.

Edinger, E. F. (1985). *Anatomy of the psyche*. Open Court.

Eliade, M. (1971). *The forge and the crucible* (S. Corrin, Trans.). Harper Torchbooks. (Original work published 1956.)

Fisher, J. V. (2019). *The uninvited guest*. Routledge.

Fordham, M. (1985). *Explorations into the self*. Karnac.

Fabricius, J. (1976). *Alchemy*. Diamond Books.

Gottman, J. S., & Gottman, J. M. (2015). *10 Principles for doing effective couples therapy*. W. W. Norton.

Greuter, M. (c. 1600). A surgery where all fantasy and follies are purged and good qualities are prescribed. [line engraving]. Wellcome Collection. https://wellcomecol lection.org/search/images?query=dpc9syce.

Grinnell, R. (1973). *Alchemy in modern woman*. Spring Publications.

Hanna, B. (1976). *Jung*. G. P. Putnam's Sons.

Hillman, J. (1975). *Re-visioning psychology*. Harper Perennial.

Hillman, J. (2014). *Alchemical psychology* (Uniform edition, vol. 5). Spring Publications.

Hollis, J. (2022). *The broken mirror*. Chiron Publications.

Toltetanus, P. (1550). *Rosarium Philosophorum*. Cyriacus Jacob. https://doi.org/10. 3931/e-rara-10570 (Original work published c. 1200s.)

Jung, C. G. (1925). Marriage as a psychological relationship. *CW* 17.

Jung, C. G. (1944). Psychology and alchemy. *CW* 12.

Jung, C. G. (1946). The psychology of the transference. *CW* 16.

Jung, C. G. (1948). General aspects of dream psychology. *CW* 8.

Jung, C. G. (1963). Mysterium coniunctionis. *CW* 14.

Jung, C. G. (1967). Alchemical studies. *CW* 13.

Jung, C. G. (1989). *Memories, dreams, reflections* (A. Jaffé, Ed.; R. Winston & C. Winston, Trans.; Rev. ed.). Vintage. (Original work published 1961.)

Kelly, E. (1893). *The alchemical writings of Edward Kelly*. James Elliott & Co. (Original work published 1676.)

Maier, M. (1617). *Symbola aureae mensae duodecim nationum*. Antonij Hummij. http s://archive.org/details/bub_gb_t_8U09S5AJ8C/mode/2up.

Maier, M. (1618). *Atalanta fugiens*. Johann-Theodor de Bry. https://digital.sciencehis tory.org/works/pc289j53n.

Maier, M. (1620). *Septimana philosophica*. Jennis. https://archive.org/details/septima naphiloso00maie/page/66/mode/2up.

Marlan, S. (2005). *The black sun*. Texas A&M University Press.

Maxwell-Stuart, P. G. (2008). *The chemical choir*. Continuum.

Moore, T. (1994). *Soul mates: Honoring the mysteries of love and relationship*. Harper Perennial.

Morgan, M. (2019). *A couple state of mind*. Routledge.

Morrison, T. (1977). *Song of Solomon*. Knopf Doubleday.

Mylius, J. D. (1622). *Philosophia reformata*. Jennis. https://doi.org/10.3931/e-rara-10756.

Mylius, J. D. (1628). *Anotomia auri*. Jennis. https://archive.org/details/joannisdanie lis00myligoog/page/n335/mode/1up.

Napier, A. Y., & Whitaker, C. (1978). *The family crucible*. Harper & Row.

Roob, A. (2021). *Alchemy & mysticism*. Taschen.

Schnarch, D. M. (1991). *Constructing the sexual crucible*. W. W. Norton & Co.

Schwartz-Salant, N. (1998). *The mystery of human relationship*. Routledge.

St. John of the Cross. (1953). *Dark night of the soul* (E. Peers, Trans.). Dover. (Original work published 1619.)

Trismosin, S. (1582). *Splendor Solis*. Kegan Paul, Trench, Trübner & Co. https://archive.org/details/SplendorSolisAlchemicalTreatisesOfSolomonTrismosin.

Tzu, L. (1988). *Tao te ching* (S. Mitchell, Trans.). Harper Perennial. (Original work published c. 400 BCE.)

von Franz, M-L. (1980). *Alchemy*. Inner City Books.

von Franz, M-L. (1990). *Psychotherapy*. Shambhala.

Winnicott, D. W. (1972). *Holding and interpretation*. Grove Press.

Chapter 7

Diversity and Contemporary Coupling

Jung's devotion to his images in night-time dreams and waking fantasies is evident throughout his *Collected Works* and fully on display in the posthumous publication of *The Red Book: Liber Novus* in 2009. He credits all his creative work to the fantasies and dreams that beset him, beginning in 1912, and began to understand the images as the expression of psychic life that arises from "the matrix of a mythopoetic imagination."[1] Dream and fantasy images reveal the life of the soul. Hillman adds that fantasy images are "the basic givens of psychic life, self-originating, inventive, spontaneous, complete, and organized in archetypal patterns. … Nothing is more primary."[2] The psyche is inherently engaged in poesis—making, imagining—in a profound creative process with individual *and* collective implications. Via imagination, the future enters "our heart, is in its innermost chamber, is in our blood," though we may not yet know what it is or how it has moved us.[3] "Only someone who is ready for everything, who doesn't exclude any experience, even the most incomprehensible," Rilke says, "will live the relationship with another person as something alive and will himself sound the depths of his own being."[4]

Why does a chapter devoted to contemporary coupling emphasize imagination? The first answer is that we are in the midst of a great cultural re-imagining of coupled life. Normative assumptions about marriage, relationship, sexuality, and gender have been questioned and dismantled by decades of critical thinking and political activism, beginning with second-wave feminism and the gay rights movement in the 1960s. Some therapists have eagerly followed and, in many instances, actively participated in these social, cultural, and political movements. They have created affirmative practices that welcome a diverse group of *queer* patients and couples: lesbian, gay, bisexual, and transgender, as well those who are nonbinary, asexual, pansexual, polyamorous, kinky, and more. This chapter draws from some of these clinicians with great appreciation for their imaginative generosity and clinical wisdom.

A second reason is that in a post-Enlightenment age, turning to the imagination and listening to the psyche is, in and of itself, a queer practice. Queer theory is multiple, fluid, and unstable[5]—not unlike the psyche. This chapter uses the verb form, *queering*, to suggest all forms of resistance to having to

DOI: 10.4324/9781032688008-8

conform to constrictive gender and sexual binaries as well as normative models of coupling. Queering, says Julie Tilson,

> is an ever-emergent process of becoming, one that is flexible and fluid in response to context, and in resistance to norms. When we queer something, we question and disrupt taken-for-granted practices and we can imagine new possibilities. Queering something breaks rules ... to liberate people who have been held hostage by what the rules require or prevent.[6]

Jung was a radically transgressive thinker in many ways, questioning and disrupting settled ideas and practices. Perhaps some of his ideas, though formulated a century ago, can find a contemporary home in queer company.

The third reason this chapter begins with the poetic imagination has to do with clinical attitude. Couples seeking professional help may be committed to an intimate relationship outside of so-called normative heterosexual, monogamous patterns of two cisgender people. A therapist's imagination must be spacious enough to envision many styles of loving so they can offer a safe, supportive, compassionate, and caring therapeutic environment. Today, the diversity of individuals and couples coming to therapy is vast, and it continues to grow.

A variety of terms and acronyms are needed to describe the diversity of contemporary couples. This chapter uses LGBTQ+ throughout. The first part of the acronym, LGBT, designates lesbian, gay, bisexual, and transgender people. The addition of Q refers to patients or couples, whether straight, lesbian, or gay, who describe themselves as *queer* when they do not identify with normative sex or gender binaries (male/female, masculine/feminine), traditional gender roles, or when they prefer to avoid labels or identities altogether. Mythically, the god at the heart of queering may well be Proteus, the shapeshifter who could rarely be grasped. The plus sign (+) at the end of LGBTQ symbolizes a fluid, open-ended way of including other designations, signaling our intention to be sensitive to the dynamic nature of this conversation. At this cultural moment, the plus sign includes N for nonbinary, I for intersex, A for asexual, and 2S, the Native American term for two-spirit people, but the list easily could grow over time to include other identities. The term *cisgender* describes the normative majority; that is, people who have the privilege of *not* thinking about gender or sexual diversity and do not face the stigma endured by LGBTQ+ people. "A cisgender person has an assigned gender that matches his/her body, a subconscious sex and gender identity that are concordant, and gender expression—ways that they show they're male or female—that's more or less conventional."[7]

Traditional norms pertaining to what it means to be in a committed relationship are also being challenged. For example, consensual nonmonogamy (CNM) is more common than many people realize. By the early 1980s (but before the AIDS crisis), CNM was the norm among gay men.[8] A 2017 study found that more than 21% of single American adults have engaged in CNM at some point and approximately 33% said they would be okay if their partner had an outside sexual relationship.[9] Curiosity about sex with multiple partners clearly has reached the cultural mainstream, even queering the two-hundred year old Regency romance, that durable bastion of heteronormative values and happily-ever-after marriage fantasies.[10] In consequence, we will use the acronym GSRD, introduced by Meg-John Barker to designate gender, sexual, or relationally diverse partners.[11] The R, which refers to those who are relationally diverse, includes straight or queer patients who have multiple partners or engage in non-normative sexuality. They may practice kink, an "umbrella term that refers generally to a range of fetish-based activities" or BDSM, which "stands for bondage and discipline, Domination and Submission, and sadism and masochism."[12]

Before going further, it is time to deconstruct the normative assumption implicit in much of psychological research and literature on couples and couples therapy: that the patients seeking therapeutic help consist of two people—a couple—in a committed relationship. This assumption is embedded in the title of our book, *The Art of Jungian* Couples *Therapy.* Earlier chapters assume that couples consist of two partners, whereas actual contemporary couples therapy sometimes includes the working out of relational dynamics among three or more intimate partners.

An Affirmative Couples Therapy

Despite the curiosity about, and existence of, alternative sexualities, severe impediments to openly claiming a queer identity or practicing kink or BDSM remain. This fact intensifies the need for affirmative therapies. Particularly in areas dominated by conservative religious views, some non-normative individuals choose to remain closeted to avoid being stigmatized or scapegoated. Best clinical practice encourages all therapists to anticipate that some of their patients will be queer-identified, which can include lesbian and gay couples, as well as partners who are transsexual, nonbinary, asexual, and consensually non-monogamous—or any of these (including straight partners) engaged in kink or BDSM. Therapists can open wider doors for couples to explore their sex lives, not by asking the usual couples intake question, *Tell me about your sex life,* but by slowing down and really inquiring, *No, really, tell me about your sex life. Everything is on the table here. It can be very important to explore what is working and what isn't.*

Because of pervasive, ongoing prejudice against LGBTQ+ people and non-normative sexual practices, couples will be looking for cues to whether it is ok to bring this material into therapy. The ongoing challenge for therapists is to examine their explicit beliefs and implicit biases and discover whether their ability to be affirming has limits. GSRD partners need compassionate witnesses for their stories. They, too, need space to explore the depths and meanings of their experiences, just like everyone else. They will be reluctant, though, if they sense that the therapist cannot receive, witness, and validate them. Or someone may be unwilling to explore sexual or gender identity issues or changes to the relationship itself—introducing kink, for instance, or consensual nonmonogamy—in front of their partner. One person's erotic fantasies may express longings of the soul that do not comfortably fit within the established relationship. In such cases, instead of pathologizing or even shaming the partner, therapists can welcome fantasies, consider them thoughtfully, and help couples negotiate new parameters for intimacy if possible.

GSRD-affirmative therapy is founded upon the clinician's ability to deeply imagine and reimagine the patient's identities (individually and as partners) and to explore any resistance to claiming an identity. It also depends upon warm, welcoming curiosity about their sexual and romantic histories, their present-day desires, and their future unlived longings—imagining the relationship *with* them in the third realm of soul. Couples therapy focused on the soul, as it is described throughout this book, *is* an affirmative therapy.

Affirmative therapies arose specifically in response to gender and sexually diverse people who face stigmatization by normative culture and to help patients navigate an LBGTQ+ identity. Affirmative therapists, according to experts in the field, do not pathologize such diversity. They understand "that the source of any pathology is rooted within a dysfunctional social context that devalues and discriminates against those who are LGBTQ+ rather than inherently within LGBTQ+ people themselves."[13] Affirmative couples therapy provides a safe container as a bulwark against social and cultural prejudice and stigma. It allows partners to discover their gender identities, sexual orientations, and patterns of loving in their own language. Partners are encouraged to speak their experience of themselves and their truth into existence—personal existence, mythic existence—through telling their deep stories. Finally, because an essential quality of soul is movement, a soul-centered affirmative therapy follows couples' movements toward embracing identities and patterns of relationship, or dancing among them, as expressions of the Self. It does not insist on one right way to be straight, lesbian, gay, bisexual, asexual, trans, nonbinary, kinky, polyamorous, and so on.

Politics in the Therapeutic Space

Until very recently in the United States, gender identities and sexual preferences other than those associated with cisgendered heterosexuality were pathologized, considered deviant, and even criminalized. (Some archaic laws are still on the books in many states.) Change and the acceptance of individual complexity has been slow in coming, with much damage done along the way to people who do not fit the normative mold. Despite efforts to create a welcoming environment, LGBTQ+ and relationally diverse patients find themselves under pressure in a polarized world that resists *queering* or destabilizing unquestioned assumptions about what is normal and natural.[14] Yet the power of eros, the sexual imagination, as well as the mystery of whom one loves and wants to live with, have always transgressed hidebound traditions.

GSRD couples often wrestle with profound psychological questions. Therapists may be called upon to help them disentangle the legacy of heteronormative role designations in order to help patients create a relationship that better suits their identities as individual partners and as a couple. Or therapists may help partners who are questioning their sexual identity, gender identity, or their preferred kind of relationship. One partner may want to explore alternative sexual practices and wonder how this emerging desire will impact the relationship. Rarely are the questions simple; most often they cut to the core of one's being. The key point is this: heteronormative social custom, cultural tradition, and the politics of LBGTQ+ identity weigh heavily on GSRD partners. The line of inquiry suggested throughout this book—*What does the soul want?*—may be especially poignant for these couples. In addition, therapists might reflect, *Does each partner feel free to follow the longings of their soul in the ways they experience love and desire?* Finally, *How can an affirmative therapist deeply listen to the hopes and anguish of partners living outside the bounds of normative relational patterns?*

The question—*What does the soul want?*—has been asked throughout this book. There is no simple answer for any troubled couple. Prevailing heteronormative assumptions make the question more fraught for GSRD patients. They are not free to love who and how they want despite political and cultural efforts to deconstruct antiquated ideas about gender, sexual identity, masculinity, and femininity, as well as so-called legitimate patterns of coupling. The ground underneath couples therapy has shifted somewhat in the last 50 years, but it has not been inclusive enough. Contending with normative assumptions about gender, sexuality, and relationships is likely to have personal—and painful—relevance for one or both partners. On this point the words of Robert Sardello are apt: "Relationships of an individual nature cannot be separated from the field of our relationships with others in the world. It is impossible to conceive of a safe haven of intimacy in a world fraught by strife and disharmony."[15] For GSRD couples, some of that strife is targeted directly at who they are, whom they love, and how they express it.

The social, political, and cultural backdrop must be kept in mind when working with GSRD couples for a simple reason: it is relevant to their experience as a couple and is likely to be an essential part of their individual stories. Your patients simply cannot grow up in the dominant culture—which takes for granted being straight, cisgender, and monogamous—without being aware of how they do not fit this mold. For example, in his affirmative practice, Douglas Thomas routinely asks patients how they have experienced themselves as *other* in familial and social milieus to explicitly acknowledge the effect of the dominant culture on LGBTQ+ people.[16]

Working with GSRD Couples

The heterosexual bias of Jungian theory is an aspect of its shadow, partly explained by historical context. Jung died in 1961, just as second-wave

feminists began challenging essentialist ideas about femininity and unquestioned beliefs about sex roles in marriage and the family. For instance, Betty
Friedan's bestselling book *The Feminine Mystique* did not appear until
1963.[17] Jung also did not live to witness gay activists demand to be seen,
accepted, and granted full political rights, which included a direct challenge
to heteronormative monogamy and procreative sexuality. Throwing out cultural scripts was (and remains) subversive and deeply unsettling, and little has
settled down since.

In 1950, when Jung presented his contrasexual theory, he introduced the
terms *anima* to describe all the characteristically feminine energies in the
psyche and *animus* for energies that have been traditionally thought of as
masculine.[18] About 30 years separate his introduction of these terms from the
1969 Stonewall Rebellion and the first Pride parade in 1970 held to honor
Stonewall.[19] This evolution made Jung's contrasexual theory an artifact of
mid-century thought, reflecting the sexual and gender binaries of its time as
well as the normative assumption that a legitimate couple consisted of one
man and one woman. While historically and culturally bound, the terms are
nonetheless quite useful when considering couples dynamics. For Jung,

> anima and animus are the archetypes of what for either sex is the totally
> other. Each represents a world that is at first quite incomprehensible to its
> opposite, a world that can never be directly known. Even though we carry
> within us elements of the opposite sex, their field of expression is precisely
> that area which is most obscure, strange, irrational, and fear-inspiring to us;
> it can at best be intuited and "felt out" but never completely understood.[20]

Part of the strange otherness of anima and animus has to do with their role as
a personification of the deepest recesses of the psyche. As mediators or go-
betweens who "filter the contents of the collective unconscious through to the
conscious mind,"[21] they take on some of the mysterious unpredictability of
the unconscious. For a cisgender man, this mediator is feminine. For a cisgender woman, the mediator is masculine.

As opposites to biological sex and conscious gender identity, the inner figures of anima and animus psychologically offer another way of being and
experiencing that are initially quite foreign. "It is normal for a man to resist
his anima," Jung says, "because she represents ... all those tendencies and
contents hitherto excluded from conscious life."[22] The same can be said about
traditional cisgender women who are comfortably held within patriarchal
culture. Her unconscious animus contains all the masculine tendencies and
contents excluded from consciousness. Resistance, however, is futile. These
contrasexual opposites may be repressed but not eradicated, and sometimes
they emerge when least expected. What does this look like? Jung asserts,
"woman is compensated by a masculine element and therefore her unconscious has, so to speak, a masculine imprint" which he calls the animus,

meaning "mind or spirit."[23] The unconscious animus, corresponding to "the paternal Logos," is characterized by "discrimination and cognition" as opposed to a woman's conscious psychological femininity, which is "characterized more by the connecting quality of Eros."[24] The animus "gives to a woman's consciousness a capacity for reflection, deliberation, and self-knowledge."[25] The anima in a man is his soul image, appearing to a young man as his mother and to an adult man as a younger woman. Often mysterious and seductive, a man's anima can express itself in "tantrums and explosive moodiness."[26] Jung also describes "the feminine" element in a man as "gushing, soulful, aesthetic, over-sensitive, etc."[27]

In practice, therapists will notice these contrasexual opposites emerging in couples' projections. Feminine-identified women, whether straight, lesbian, or queer, will project their less-conscious masculinity onto the men in their lives, including fathers, brothers, partners, and others. Similarly, masculine-identified men, whether straight, gay, or queer, project their femininity onto mothers, sisters, partners, and others. By contrast, a masculine-identified woman will project femininity onto opposite-sex others and a feminine-identified man will project masculinity onto opposite-sex others.

Marie-Louise von Franz, Jung's long-time collaborator and biographer, offers this precise summary:

> The anima comprises the positive and negative—for the most part also repressed—feminine characteristics in a man. In its positive aspect, it is feminine empathy or sensitivity, sometimes also the sense of feeling, eros, artistic tendencies, love of nature, acceptance of the validity of the irrational. Negatively, it is moodiness, irritability, subjective judgment, whininess, hypochondria, and sentimentality. The animus in a woman manifests positively as initiative, depth of thought, consistency, courage, sense of religious truth; negatively as rigid opinionatedness, brutality, exaggeratedly masculine behavior, and so on.[28]

These statements by Jung and von Franz assume that *femininity* and *masculinity* are stable, uncontested categories. Further, they assume that a woman is ego-identified with femininity and a man is ego-identified with masculinity. They do not question their meanings or their assignment, masculinity to men, femininity to women. Feminist and archetypal theory does question both meaning and assignment and, in the spirit of this chapter, queers the categories.

In addition to its application to relational dynamics, Jung's contrasexual theory of animus and anima also provides useful ways of thinking about the individuation process for couples. When therapists notice one partner projecting their gender opposite, anima or animus, onto the other, it is an opportunity to examine, psychologically, what is being displaced or disowned. Fundamentally, the aim of reclaiming inner masculine and feminine figures is movement toward wholeness, sometimes symbolized as psychological androgyny. Psychological androgyny was a radical idea in 1950 when Jung first published his theory, and it remains radical today. The term itself is apparently threatening to the ego, despite the numerous creation stories that identify androgyny as the primal undifferentiated unity from which the earliest divisions occur.[29]

Excursion: Anima as Soul

A key concern of soul-centered therapy must address itself to Jung's conflation of anima, the inner feminine possessed only by men, and soul. According to classical Jungian theory, women did not have an anima. They only possessed an animus—defined as spirit, not soul—which dissatisfied many of Jung's female students and patients.[30] Instead, women themselves were regarded as soul figures *for men*.

Yet here is a curiosity relevant to couples therapy: the description of the anima offered by von Franz could easily suggest the soul's participation in intimate relationship for men, women, or nonbinary persons. The reader need only ignore the male pronouns. "She [anima] represents the flow of life in a man's psyche. He has to follow up its tortuous ways, which move very specifically just between the two borders of inside and outside."[31] Therapists are frequent witnesses to the tortuous ways of relationships. Partners typically enter therapy when the suffering becomes unbearable.

The multiplicity and variability of inner figures emphasized by archetypal psychology assert that anyone, regardless of sex or gender, can discover their feminine anima among the innumerable psychic persons in the unconscious.[32] She presents herself disguised as an "endless variety of figures" reflecting "the endlessness of the soul."[33] Wholeness for any of us, then, consists in welcoming anima figures as soul images, who guide us in the unique and intimate process of soul-making.

Jung has been justly criticized for the obvious essentialism and misogyny in his theory of contrasexual archetypes.[34] Particularly concerning, says Susan Rowland, is Jung's tendency to collapse gender identity into bodily sex. A product of his time, he believed that "body shape bestowed a straightforward gender identity on women and men," an attitude that "leads to innate femininity and masculinity."[35] But Rowland also notes that Jung's bodily essentialism is tempered by the fluidity of concepts such as femininity and masculinity and by his contrasexual theory. That is, Jungian theory asserts that none of us is exclusively masculine or feminine, irrespective of sexual identity, gender identity, or who and how we love. Therapists honor the psyche's natural multiplicity and fluidity in service of individuation, helping couples discover and accept the multiple aspects of their character. It is fundamentally an inclusive endeavor.

Nonetheless, there remain therapists who maintain a rigid understanding of sexual and gender binaries and do considerable harm when they perpetuate the kinds of prejudice and stigma that queer patients and couples continue to face in the social environment. As queer-affirming training programs and queer-affirming clinicians and scholars continue to peel away heteronormative cultural encrustations, Jung's contrasexual theory, which is fluid and context-sensitive, will remain generative for therapists working with straight cisgender and queer partners.

Couples and Gender Roles

A foundational idea running through Jung's work is the notion of holding the tension of the opposites. Opposites, and the tension they create, is evident throughout Jung's formulations of typology (Chapter 4) and the shadow (Chapter 5). It shows up in couples therapy in the fantasy *you complete me*, the idea that the partner's complementary attributes form a whole, together, instead of each person striving toward individual wholeness. In any kind of a relationship, partners unconsciously project their contrasexual opposite onto each other, rather than recognizing it as part of their own identity. This is readily observed clinically when, for example, a wife demands that her husband take care of finances and discipline the kids, or when a husband expects his wife to cook, clean, and be the nurturing presence by carrying the emotional life of the family. Daily living with contrasexual projections is an inestimable opportunity to see, in an embodied form, one's inner gender opposite.

It is difficult to take back one's projected psychic material. Couples therapists know that these projections are very sticky. But with patient, persistent, psychological discernment, partners can begin to see the qualities and capacities they have unconsciously given to their partner and, by retrieving them, gain access to their fuller Selves. For example, after listening to the tearful expression of one partner, a therapist, noticing the flat affect of the other partner, can turn to them and say, *That was really sad to hear. I'm wondering where your tears are, your sadness, your deep feelings about this matter? Do you notice that your partner is carrying the emotions for both of you?* The therapist may need to wait for a response, particularly when the partner doesn't *do* emotion—that is, when they have projected emotional expression onto the other. The therapist might continue *I know you have deep feelings about this. I'm feeling them myself! If you can share some of your emotions around this, it will be easier for your partner. They will not feel alone in it, and both of you will feel better, even if nothing changes.*

The value of thinking in opposites persists regardless of whether one or both partners identify as cisgender or nonbinary. Moreover, therapists need not literalize contrasexual figures. Instead, they can imagine the underlying energies of anima and animus flowing (or not) between the partners regardless of sex or gender identity. The opposites, as symbolic markers of difference, can help a couple sort out their psychological identities by growing curious about how *this is not like that* in their inner world. Re-imagining gender roles and sexual identities as loosely held modes of being makes the fullness of human experience equally available to cis-gender partners as well as queer individuals.

For example, when codified gender and sexual identity roles and rules no longer fit for couples, therapists can help explore the meaning that partners assign to *feminine* and *masculine* by inviting them to imagine their personal associations to those terms, possibly using language or playing with gesture, posture, facial expression, or movement. They could ask partners to embody their understanding of femininity. What emerges? They could do the same with masculinity, and again, notice what emerges. Therapists might also invite couples to bring dream images to sessions and pay attention when the figures are strongly gendered or not. They can help couples discuss when and how they distribute so-called feminine and masculine roles or behaviors on a day-to-day basis—and also how they queer such roles as a way to honor the fullness of both types of energies in each partner.

Anima and Animus in the Twenty-first Century

Jung was the first psychologist "to postulate a bisexual complexity at the heart of every individual."[36] At the time, the very idea that men had an inner feminine and women an inner masculine radically destabilized traditional gender norms, the implications of which are still reverberating today. As Tacey asserts, "Jung's theory of our contrasexual nature remains invaluable to our understanding of development, and our task is to retrieve the theory from its sexism so that we can do justice to the gender diversity that is valued today."[37]

Instead of oppositions—cisgender females paired with an inner masculine (the animus) or cisgender males paired with an inner feminine (the anima)—affirmative therapy with couples works with the entire host of figures alive in each partner's inner world. These inner figures can spontaneously appear in many forms and guises, including female, male, androgyne, human, and more-than-human. The figures are drawn from ancient myth, contemporary fiction, the partner's own ancestry, and other ancestors outside of their literal bloodline and inherited cultures. When such figures show up in dreams, fantasies, reveries, via a felt sense of their presence, or in dialogue, therapists can greet them with warm interest and curiosity to help couples work with the animus and anima energies they embody.

This emphasis on multiplicity supports contemporary ideas of gender fluidity. Individuation, as the path toward wholeness, may not be an encounter with one inner figure who is clearly masculine or feminine. Instead, it may involve welcoming multiple inner figures who exceed the bounds of any sex or gender category. Partners, regardless of gender or sexual identity, can discover many ways of expressing both their feminine and masculine energies. Queering the categories *feminine* and *masculine* is a way to play with the normative rules and roles of relationship. When partners do fall into normative roles—and it becomes constricting for them—therapists can encourage them to imagine other ways of being.

Transgression and the Soul of Relationship

Some GSRD couples may feel the pull to non-normative relationships as an aspect of "the soul's transgressive necessity," the subtitle of Thomas' important 2023 work on BDSM and kink. These "intentionally transgressive sexualities" cause many people to recoil, including therapists, yet a surprising number of people do the opposite: then lean in, become curious, and imagine it for themselves. "The general public appears to be both tantalized and misinformed about the details of BDSM culture."[38] Thomas notes three important themes in work with GSRD couples, whether the partners practice kink or not.

First, Thomas notes "a *telos* or deeper purpose that is drawing people forward in their individuation process."[39] Alternate sexualities—as well as alternate gender identities and being in a GSRD relationship—may be a spiritual calling and a soul necessity, fundamental to a partner's wholeness. Therapists help GSRD couples listen for this calling and use an expansive imagination to help partners embody and accept more of who they are. If such a calling puts pressure on a relationship, therapists can support a couple as they negotiate these sometimes-incompatible needs.

Second, partners who practice kink, or who engage in CNM, polyamory, and other erotic combinations in an ethical manner, need to communicate with each other clearly, honestly, and frequently. Good communication is essential to ethical alternate sexualities. BDSM and kink rest on an "elaborate process of negotiation and consent"[40]—and require a level of consciousness about roles and responsibilities within the relationship—that straight or LGBTQ+ couples would benefit from emulating.

Third, in Thomas' epilogue, *love* is the final word. The dictionary definition of love, he says, is "a reasonable starting place yet wholly unsatisfactory" because

> it misses the quality of poetic expansion that love brings to life. It misses the ecstatic longing, the mystery, and the madness, too. It is the irrational aspect of love that brings it into relationship with soul. Love, like soul … is a deliberately ambiguous concept—its multifaceted power stems from this ambiguity. We pretend to understand it as a primordial force that is living through us, but at root, it is a mystery.[41]

Love is the final word in affirmative couples therapy, too, where therapists welcome each LBGTQ+ person and GSRD couple, greeting their identities and desires with respect and full clinical curiosity. If therapists can remain open, they witness the same expressions of archetypal longing, mystery, and madness they see in their work with straight couples. It is a queer practice in all the best senses of that word.

Queering Your Therapy Practice

Tilson encourages therapists to queer their practice.[42] There are many ethical reasons for doing so since the broad aim of an affirmative therapy for GSRD couples is to offer them what they frequently do not receive in social situations: visibility and acceptance of who they are and who they are becoming in the life-long process of individuation together. Tilson's four step outline for affirmative therapy with individuals also works for couples.[43] First, engage with curiosity about how partners make meaning of gender, sexuality, relationships, and identity. Second, help partners place their stories in the context of cultural narratives, which none of us can entirely escape. Tilson refers to this as "listening to the world in the room."[44] Third, consider multiple possible understandings of their stories. Finally, situate the stories, and the meanings partners make of them, in specific contexts. Rather than universalize their stories, particularize them.

Some of the complexities that can arise with GSRD couples include multiple and conflicting stories, experiences, and meanings. One partner in an LGBTQ+ relationship may be more out to friends, colleagues, and family than the other, or face more discrimination at work. One partner may resist identifying themselves, not wanting to be categorized or labeled, which their partner might interpret as rejection or internalized homophobia. Some partners are concerned about how they present, when and for whom: their social persona as a couple. Since that couple persona can fluctuate depending upon context, they may disagree about how to present in specific situations—an office party, for instance, or a family wedding—and what the presentation means about their relationship. One partner may be bisexual, not homosexual, or seeking a kinkier sex life, or feel they need to transition to embody a more congruent identity. Of course, every one of these issues, and many more, affects *both* partners and the relationship. Added to these tensions are all the typical issues that beset couples generally: struggles over communication, money, home life, sex life, raising children, and taking care of elders. Even seemingly enjoyable activities such as hosting a party or planning vacations together can be fraught.

Listening to a couple's stories with a generous heart is an active, engaged praxis. It may be more like dialogue as therapists ask questions, probe for elusive, significant details, note moments of surprise or shifts in understanding, or when a couple struggles to imagine something different. Tilson admits, "This is an experience that I hear from many trans and nonbinary people. They feel adrift, and are often in significant distress, until they encounter the language that helps them speak themselves into the world."[45] Often, therapists will need to slow down the conversation to encourage couples to pay attention to their own words—and the words of their partner.

Yet therapists must be careful not to inject language, especially labels, into their work with couples in an effort to be helpful. Virginia Satir's reminder to therapists to "lead from a half-step behind" encourages the partners to take the lead, step into their power, follow their own images, and discover their own meanings.[46] Therapists bear witness to partners as they speak themselves into the world and includes listening to their suffering, both past and present, all the while remaining attuned to what the soul wants.[47] Sometimes a story "is so resonant, so right, it causes us to remember, at least for an instant, what substance we are really made from, and where is our true home."[48] Evoking such stories may begin a subtle process of repair for a suffering couple. As intimated in Chapter 3, the untold story may contain its own remedy.

Telling the untold story may be especially meaningful for GSRD couples because they, too, are in search of stories they can live in, stories that fit better for who they actually are, stories that express their unfathomed depths as a couple as well as nurturing their individual lives. In Christine Downing's book on same-sex love, she argues that "by and large we have been the defined not the self-definers, the objects of others' mythmaking rather than the creators of our own mythology."[49] She sustains hope that by exploring "the various histories, the various stories, the various myths" by and about LGBTQ+ people (and couples), "we may see more clearly where each of us would want to insist on differences, where each would be ready to affirm similarities."[50] Sharing therapeutic space with an affirming therapist attuned to the myths and mysteries of eros is a welcome relief. As Tilson and Nichols point out, a couple's issues may have little or nothing to do with their GSRD identity, but they are unlikely to stay and do the deep work they came to do unless they feel welcome and accepted.[51]

Self-reflexivity, Countertransference, and Fragility

Earlier chapters describe the critical importance of the transferential field in therapy. Hillman describes the transference as "a unique relationship together with all its complicated expectations about their joint destiny" in which therapists are "involved in the other's life as no one else is."[52] Therapists may not like to admit it, but couples do become involved in the therapist's psychic life—not in terms of social knowledge, though some facts about the therapist's life will undoubtedly come out over time—but through the interpenetration of unconscious contents. It is a relationship of "mutual influence, in which the whole being of the doctor as well as the patient plays its part."[53] A partner or couple will mean something to the therapist personally, "which provides the most favourable basis for treatment."[54] Moreover, no matter how many years of experience therapists have, they "will discover again and again" that they are "caught up in a bond ... resting on mutual unconsciousness."[55]

The persistence of unconsciousness—Jung's assertion that we are forever dogged by what we do not know about ourselves including our assumptions, biases, and beliefs—can quickly come to the consciousness of therapists working with LGBTQ+ partners and relationally diverse couples in general. Possibly for the first time, therapists will have to face their own discomfort with queerness in any of its multifaceted expressions, ask themselves about the meanings of normality, or realize their current limits of acceptance and compassion. The transferential field "is the root of analysis" and "the living symbol of the healing process" that expresses its "continually changing and gripping eros."[56] GSRD partners may go more deeply into those dark roots than any other, and take the therapist with them.

Psychoanalyst Annie Rogers, says this about the therapeutic relationship:

> Each person brings to that relationship whatever is unrecognized, unknown, the unapproachable in her or his life, and a wish for knowledge of truths and wholeness. Since one cannot thrive on memories, on a relationship with projections, what keeps alive the hope of wholeness is an interchange of love, longing, frustration, and anger in the vicissitudes of a real relationship. Such an interchange is part of the fragility of this relationship; with openness, one is vulnerable to hurt and to loss, on both sides of the relationship.[57]

Many contemporary partners—whether straight or GSRD—long for a "real relationship" regardless of its frustrations and vicissitudes. Even if they live in deeply conservative geographical areas, many now have access to parts of a wider world where some of the traditional parameters for committed relationships have been questioned, eroded, or rejected. Couples are likely to arrive for therapy with more options for how to be a couple, more freedom to choose, and also more confusion. Rogers' observation about the fragility of relationships is true for therapeutic relationships, for the suffering partners, and perhaps for all of us at a time when so many constricting customs and structures, once taken for granted, are vigorously debated. For queer theorists and GSRD affirmative therapists, any broadening of perspective is a welcome change, but working in such a fluid context is nonetheless a psychological challenge.

Therapists as well as researchers are well-versed in the importance of self-knowledge, a theme reiterated throughout *The Art of Jungian Couples Therapy*. In psychological literature the pursuit of self-knowledge is referred to as *self-reflexivity* and sometimes as *positionality*. Fundamentally, both concepts mean that each of us "speaks from a particular class, gendered, racial, cultural, and ethnic community perspective" who "approaches the world with a set of ideas, a framework (theory, ontology) that specifies a set of questions (epistemology)."[58] Self-reflexivity goes beyond mere reverie or reflection. It is the therapist's active effort to probe when, how, and why they were affected by the therapeutic work. For instance, *What did the uncomfortable moments with a couple reveal about my beliefs or assumptions? How do my values prevent me from opening more fully to a couple? If I want to be more affirmative, how can I educate myself? Can I explore biases, implicit or otherwise, with colleagues or in supervision? If I am unable to meet a couple where they are, can I limit damage and refer them out?*

Self-reflexivity in a Jungian mode obligates therapists to probe more deeply. Examining inherited social, cultural, and religious beliefs, as well as their identities conferred by class, sex, ethnicity, education, and age is not enough. A Jungian perspective also asks therapists to recognize their own unconscious complexes when they are activated—or shortly thereafter. It takes great presence of mind and psychological poise to do so. Not doing so, being unaware of activated complexes, interferes with an open and accepting clinical attitude. As Chapter 2's discussion of complexes made clear, an activated complex can derail even the most well-intentioned couples therapist.

Conclusion

Since there are no *right ways* to be partners or *right kinds* of partnership, affirmative therapists witness the movements of eros between people as lively, mutable, and fascinating expressions of their souls. Archetypal multiplicity is a direct outgrowth of Jungian theory, yet it is far different from Jung's traditional twentieth-century views of sex and gender. Part of the individuation process relevant in today's queer, gender-fluid world is first recognizing, accepting, and working with one's own multiplicity regardless of gender or sexual identity.

Affirmative practice expands therapeutic perspectives to flexibly support the varieties of coupling experience. Archetypal patterns (see Chapter 3) gain their psychological usefulness in how they are fleshed out by partners in relationship, which is always contextual. Coupling itself is an archetypal pattern. Who couples, how they form the partnership, and what values, beliefs, desires, and behaviors support their life together are culturally (and individually) specific. Cultural customs and beliefs exist, but affirmative therapy does not support a coercive, reductive, normative script for the multifaceted expressions of eros. Indeed, eros is a formidable power and a great mystery to be ever-lived and explored.

In a passage with particular relevance to therapists working with GSRD couples, Jung asserts the influence of therapy beyond its benefits to the suffering partners: "The bond established by the transference," as confusing and difficult as it may be, "is vitally important not only for the individual but also for society, and indeed for the moral and spiritual progress of mankind."[59] The therapist "is not just working for this particular patient [or couple] ... but for himself as well as his own soul."[60] Moreover, Jung adds, therapists are engaged in cultural work, because "the ultimate questions of psychotherapy are not a private matter—they represent a supreme responsibility."[61]

In a polarized moment when powerful social, religious, and political forces are arrayed against LGBTQ+ people and nonnormative couples relationships, contributions by affirmative couples therapists are a supreme responsibility. An expansive approach to GSRD partners, focused on the soul, is fundamentally generous. Who can know how, when, and where such therapists might tip the balance in favor of love?

Notes

1 Jung 1989[1961], p. 188.
2 Hillman 1975, p. xvii.

3 Rilke 2021, p. 66.
4 Rilke 1993, p. 98.
5 See the excellent classical works in the field by Jagose 1996 and Sedgwick 1990.
6 Tilson 2021, p. 6.
7 Nichols 2021, p.183.
8 Nichols 2021, pp. 279–280.
9 Nichols 2021, pp. 279–280.
10 For example, *Bridgerton* (Beers et al. 2021), the massively popular Regency romance streaming on Netflix, strongly favors the happily-ever-after trope of married monogamy typical of the genre. However, it also queered the Romance in Season 3 by dramatizing multiple consensual erotic scenes with two men and one woman. Similarly, the overwhelming popularity of *Fifty Shades of Grey* (James 2015) attests to mainstream fascination with kink.
11 Barker 2019.
12 Thomas 2023, p. xvii.
13 Harvey et al. 2012, p. 18.
14 As Nichols (2021) points out, political and religious forces have attempted to turn back the clock to a time when straight, cisgender couples in monogamous marriages, whose sexual activity aimed at procreation rather than pleasure, prevailed. This conservative fantasy has never fully described human relationships or sexualities.
15 Sardello 1995, p. 162.
16 Thomas 2023.
17 Friedan 1963.
18 Jung's writings on *anima* and *animus* were published in 1950 by the Analytical Psychology Club of New York and are included in Volumes 7 (1953) and 9ii (1959) of his *Collected Works*.
19 The Stonewall rebellion was a spontaneous uprising that took place at a gay club in Greenwich Village, New York City, on June 28th 1969, marking a new era to claim political rights. The 50th anniversary of Stonewall in 2019 demonstrated that the fight is long, arduous, and continues. While there have been significant gains in some parts of the world, backlash and repression are equally evident. Backlash against the gains of second-wave feminism are equally stark, evidenced by the 2022 repudiation of the landmark Supreme Court decision known as *Roe v. Wade*.
20 Whitmont 1979, p. 185.
21 Jung 1959, para. 40.
22 Jung 1940, para. 129.
23 Jung 1959, para. 29.
24 Jung 1959, para. 29.
25 Jung 1959, para. 33.
26 Jung 1953, para. 319.
27 Jung 1928, para. 220.
28 von Franz 1999, p. 364.
29 Eliade 1960.
30 Downing 1988, p. 138.
31 von Franz 1970, p. 68.
32 Hillman 1975.
33 Hillman 1979, p. 41.
34 Cf. Goldenberg 1990, Lauter & Ruprecht 1985, Rowland 2002, and Wehr 1987.
35 Rowland 2002, p. 32.
36 Tacey 2012, p. 144.
37 Tacey 2012, pp. 145–146.

38 Thomas 2023, p. 11.
39 Thomas 2023, p. xix.
40 Thomas 2023, p. 11.
41 Thomas 2023, p. 248.
42 Tilson 2021.
43 Tilson 2021, pp. 22–23.
44 Tilson 2021, p. 34.
45 Tilson 2021, p. 35.
46 Satir 2001.
47 Glassman 1988.
48 Pinkola-Estes 1992, p. 7.
49 Downing 1989, p. 3.
50 Downing 1989, p. 11.
51 See Tilson 2021 and Nichols 2021.
52 Hillman 1997, p. 19.
53 Jung 1946, para. 163.
54 Jung 1946, para. 365.
55 Jung 1946, para. 367.
56 Hillman 1997, p. 19.
57 Rogers 1995, p. 319.
58 Denzin & Lincoln 2011, p. 11.
59 Jung 1946, para. 449.
60 Jung 1946, para. 449.
61 Jung 1946, para. 449.

References

Barker, M. (2019). *Gender, sexual, and relationship diversity (GSRD)*. BACP House.
Beers, B., Rhimes, S. Robinson, J. & van Dusen, C. (2021–present). *Bridgerton*. [TV series] Netflix. https://www.netflix.com.
Denzin, N. & Lincoln, Y. (2011). Introduction: The discipline and practice of qualitative research. In *The Sage handbook of qualitative research* (4th ed., pp. 1–20). Sage.
Downing, C. (1988). *Psyche's sisters*. Harper & Row.
Downing, C.(1989). *Myths and mysteries of same-sex love*. Continuum.
Eliade, M. (1960). *Myths, dreams, and mysteries*. Harper Torchbooks.
Friedan, B. (1963). *The feminine mystique*. W. W. Norton & Co.
Glassman, B. (1988). *Bearing witness*. Harmony.
Goldenberg, N. (1990). A feminist critique of Jung. In *Jung and Christianity in dialog* (R. Moore & D. Meckel, Eds.). Paulist Press.
Harvey, R., Murphy, M. J., Bigner, J. J., & Wetchler, J. L. (Eds.). (2012). *Handbook of LGBTQ-affirmative couple and family therapy* (2nd ed.). Routledge.
Hillman, J. (1975). *Re-visioning psychology*. HarperPerennial.
Hillman, J. (1979). *The dream and the underworld*. Harper & Row.
Hillman, J. (1985). *Anima, An anatomy of a personified notion*. Spring Publications.
Hillman, J. (1997). *Suicide and the soul* (2nd ed.). Spring Publications.
Jagose, A. (1996). *Queer theory: An introduction*. New York University Press.
James, E. L. (2015). *Fifty shades of grey*. Vintage Books.
Jung, C. G. (1928). The love problem of a student. *CW* 10.
Jung, C. G. (1940). Psychology and religion: West and east. *CW* 11.

Jung, C. G. (1946). The psychology of the transference. *CW* 16.

Jung, C. G. (1953). Two essays in analytical psychology. *CW* 7.

Jung, C. G. (1959). Aion. *CW* 9ii.

Jung, C. G. (1989). *Memories, dreams, reflections* (A. Jaffé, Ed.; R. Winston & C. Winston, Trans.; Rev. ed.). Vintage. (Original work published 1961.)

Jung, C. G. (2009). *Liber novus[The red book]*. S. Shamdasani (Ed.) (M. Kyburz, J. Peck, & S. Shamdasani, Trans.). W. W. Norton & Co.

Lauter, E., & Ruprecht, C. (Eds.). (1985). *Feminist archetypal theory.* University of Tennessee Press.

Nichols, M. (2021). *The modern clinician's guide to working with LGBTQ+ clients.* Routledge.

Pinkola-Estes, C. (1992). *Women who run with the wolves.* Ballantine Books.

Rilke, R. M. (1993). *Letters to a young poet* (S. Mitchell, Trans.). Shambhala.

Rilke, R. M.(2021). *Letter to a young poet* (A. Barrows & J. Macy, Trans.) Shambhala.

Rogers, A. (1995). *A Shining affliction.* Penguin.

Rowland, S. (2002). *Jung, a feminist revision.* Routledge.

Satir, V. (2001). *Virginia Satir: Foundational ideas* (B. J. Brothers, Ed.). Routledge.

Sardello, R. (1995). *Love and the soul.* HarperCollins.

Sedgwick, E. (1990). *Epistemology of the closet.* Berkeley: University of California Press.

Tacey, D. (2012). *The essential Jung.* Routledge.

Thomas, D. (2023). *The deep psychology of BDSM and kink.* Routledge.

Tilson, J. (2021). *Queering your therapy practice.* Routledge.

Wehr, D. (1987). *Jung and feminism.* Beacon Press.

Whitmont, E. (1979). *The symbolic quest.* Princeton University Press.

von Franz, M.-L. (1970). *An introduction to the psychology of fairy tales.* Spring Publications.

von Franz, M.-L. (1999). *Archetypal dimensions of the psyche.* Shambhala.

Chapter 8

Jung and the Soul of the Therapist

"Psychotherapy is an unidentified technique applied to unspecified circumstances with unpredictable outcomes. For this technique, we recommend rigorous training."[1] Such was the infamous declaration some years ago, overheard at a psychotherapy conference. It begs the question: What draws therapists to such a challenging profession? There are certainly (much) easier ways to earn a (better) living that require (much) less education and training. This chapter poses important personal questions using the mythic, archetypal, soulful perspective infusing the entire book: *What soul wounds brought you to this work? What archetypal constellations shape your life? What myths or fairy tales have you in their grips? What alchemical gold are you seeking?* We invite you to return periodically to these questions to help uncover more of the unconscious forces influencing your approach to clinical work and life because few other professions place such intense demands on the soul. This chapter focuses on the need for therapists to tend their own souls, both during and outside of sessions.

There are at least two reasons therapists must prioritize tending their own souls. First, the sheer intensity of transference energies between partners and between couples and the therapist affects therapists at the deepest levels of their psyches. Partners transfer their conscious and unconscious contents onto and into each other *and* the therapist. In turn, the therapist experiences countertransference, projecting their unconscious contents onto partners and their relationship. Fundamentally, this means that therapists are drawn into the depths of the couple's unfolding drama, whether they want to be or not. A couple's distress compels participation, which undermines the therapist's efforts to maintain a degree of neutrality.

Second, therapists need to tend their own souls because the experience of couples therapy is intimate and alive. It cannot help but stir painful personal memories, wounds, and fantasies about love, relationships, and commitment. The therapeutic container, highly charged particularly when working with couples, places higher psychic demands on therapists. The need to tend their own soul, for its own sake, is an integral part of the work that goes beyond good advice about self-care[2] and the therapist's use of self.[3] Cultivating an ongoing

DOI: 10.4324/9781032688008-9

relationship with one's unconscious by engaging with inner images, figures, dreams, and reveries for the sake of individuation is soul work.

Asking therapists immersed in a helping profession to care for their own souls often runs counter to their inclinations. The constellation of a helping or healing archetype often comes at the expense of honoring one's Self and, whether acknowledged or not, creates a power differential in the consulting room.[4] Over time, therapists' efforts to help others often become not selfless but Self-less. That is, there is a tendency to quit caring for one's Self in the false belief that doing so is selfish. Yet without the Self, therapists have nothing to work with because the totality of the therapist *is* the attuning instrument in the consulting room. To work in the depths with couples, therapists must remain attuned to their own depths, moment over clinical moment, as an act of service. Rachel Naomi Remen elaborates:

> Helping, fixing, and serving represent three different ways of seeing life. When you help, you see life as weak. When you fix, you see life as broken. When you serve, you see life as whole. Fixing and helping may be the work of the ego, and service the work of the soul.[5]

Therapists contend with considerable amounts of anxiety and insecurity as they face the unknown with struggling couples. Since they are working day in and day out with soul in all its many forms, a Jungian approach invites therapists to become students of soul. But manualizing a Jungian approach to couples therapy would insult the totality of the psyches in the consulting room, the therapist's and the couple's. Jung describes how he worked: "I put my patients in front of me and I talk to them as one natural human being to another, and I expose myself completely and react with no restriction."[6] However, the degree of vulnerability Jung describes does not imply a wild analysis,[7] nor should it be forgotten that the foundation of Jung's clinical work was his ongoing, robust relationship with his own inner world, his own soul. Rather, the art of couples therapy lies in creating a holding container that is both sturdy and porous, a space in which you and the couple listen for soul. Tending your own soul is essential to maintaining this degree of vulnerability.

Therapists, like the holding container, also need to be emotionally, spiritually, and imaginally porous because "you can exert no influence if you are not susceptible to influence."[8] But Jungian analyst David Sedgwick cautions that therapy "is not a platform for spontaneous expression, whether that be general pontification on various matters, including a patient's [or couple's] life-choices, or discussing his or others' life or problems."[9] An intentionally well-crafted and well-boundaried therapeutic container invites all psyches into a co-constructed, live, emergent space, allowing for an expansion of consciousness and movement toward healing.[10] Ultimately, therapists continually tend their own soul because "one cannot help any patient to advance further than one has advanced oneself."[11]

Soul and Self

Jung had much to say about the impact the practice of therapy has on the therapist. Contemporary advances in neuroscience have verified much of what he formulated.[12] The meandering, non-linear ways of psyche, Self, and soul are usually the first casualties in standardized training for therapists. But couples therapists are quickly reminded of the mystery of relationships when confronted with real, live, hurting (and hurtful) partners. The clinical ground of being can suddenly evaporate in a charged environment, rendering clinical training ineffectual. Manualized approaches may be met with dead eyes, worksheets lose meaning, and prescriptives go unheeded. Therapists feeling such powerlessness in the face of live complexes (see Chapter 2) may instinctively reach for their protective clinical armor. Instead, we invite you to proactively shed the armor, forego a fix-it approach, and choose psychological vulnerability and curiosity.

Continually moving toward discomfort and uncertainty is difficult. And yet, to bring a more authentic Self into the consulting room, couples therapists must first become more familiar *and* comfortable with that Self. This includes not only acknowledging their inherent shortcomings, blind spots, woundings, fears, weaknesses, imperfections, and limitations but actually moving toward them with curiosity, nonjudgmental regard and, ultimately, acceptance. Therapists, no matter how much personal therapy they have done, can patiently notice the ongoing nature of the process itself.

"In antiquity the physician healed through his own suffering," says Hillman, adding that "the wound that would not heal was the well of cures."[13] Life's big wounds, or *soul wounds*, never heal completely, nor should they. Tending your own soul is tending these wounds. By staying close to your deep wounding, you also stay close to *your* well of cures.

Soul and Method

Jung cautions, "the enormous increase of technical facilities only serves to occupy the mind with all sorts of sensations and impressions that lure the attention and interest from the inner world."[14] In daily practice, therapists must approach sessions by "leaving aside all theory and listening attentively" rather than trying to learn "recipes by heart and then apply them more or less suitably."[15] Yet when faced with the unknown in the consulting room, therapists often search from among the ever-growing number of treatment modalities and trainings to ease professional anxieties. As the clinician's focus shifts outward, the intimate matters of the soul are obscured.

The vocation of couples therapy invites therapists into the mystery of relationships: *What is going on here between these two people?* In search of answers, therapists can follow Wilfred Bion in cultivating a not-knowing clinical stance.[16] Theoretical physicist Fred Alan Wolf also reminds us, "The real trick to life is not to be in the know, but to be in the mystery."[17] Therapists can actively observe their internal back-and-forth movement between knowing and not-knowing (a saturated and unsaturated mind) while inviting couples to do the same. Fostering perpetual curiosity requires dissolving clinical judgments, perceptions, and theory almost as quickly as they form in the mind, allowing way to lead on to way, as the poet Robert Frost intimates.[18]

Jung places the whole of the therapist fully in the consulting room and the therapeutic relationship, noting, "one is naturally loath to admit that one could be affected in the most personal way by just any patient [or couple]."[19] Because of the mutual alchemy of transference, therapists are not just *doing therapy* with couples; the therapy alters them, too. Sedgwick cautions that therapists remain aware of their "professional responsibility, expertise, and role" while also knowing they are in "a more vulnerable position vis-à-vis the patient and vis-à-vis his own unconscious as affected by the patient [or couple]."[20] Adding, "Jung was adamant, almost to the point of role reversal, about the therapist and the patient meeting on these equal psychological terms, and he was highly critical of a therapist's escaping this by hiding behind a professional persona."[21]

Therapists who closely follow how the work is altering them are tending soul and its movement. Sedgwick adds:

> Psychotherapy is therefore an act of emotional involvement, self-understanding, and healing for the Jungian [couples] therapist as well as for the Jungian patient[s]. In the course of responding to the contagious complexes of the patient [or couple], the therapist's reactions and processes form the backbone of the work. Not only does the patient discover his feelings, the therapist discovers his.[22]

Yet, with almost complete emphasis on training and technique as well as sole focus on the couple's psychological process, a therapist can easily forget or ignore the profound impact on the Self.

The following personal anecdote (Delmedico) highlights this impact. Early in individual therapy, I confronted my therapist, telling them that they could stop with the faux empathy, exclaiming that they did not really care about me and that the moment I quit paying, they would quickly forget me. Aside from an indicator of some of the work that lay ahead for us, I clearly had no idea how the therapeutic encounter affects the therapist. Therapists know this is not a *fee for empathy* business, nor are patients merely renting space in the therapist's mind for a clinical hour. In fact, the whole of the therapist cannot un-know the experience of the other. Whether consciously or unconsciously, patients do not rent space, they take up permanent residence in the therapist. Clinical experience alters who therapists are. Despite seeming to *forget* a couple between sessions or after termination, it can all come rushing back in a moment of reverie or when a couple returns, sometimes years later.

The deep psyche knows and remembers. Therapists are in the work with couples, whether they want to be or not.

When Jo Wheelwright was trying to found one of the first Jungian training institutes in the United States, Jung told him, "Why don't you try and have the most disorganized organization you can manage?"[23] Jung knew that overreliance on theoretical knowledge and institutional constraints fetters the therapist's psyche, and he wanted to avoid making dogma out of his work. "Thank God I am Jung, and not a Jungian!,"[24] he once exclaimed, wholly disinterested in creating a group of therapists who *did it* like him. Joseph Campbell also stresses individuation, saying, "The privilege of a lifetime is being who you are," an imperative that is particularly applicable in the practice of therapy.[25] Very few professions, if any, work so deeply, so intensely, and for so long with the psyche. Hour over (sometimes excruciating) clinical hour, over years and decades, therapists confront and reevaluate their previously held beliefs, fears, hopes—all their ideas about who we are as humans, both individually and collectively. Authentic presence forces therapists away from *holding it all tightly together* to being somewhat loosely held together in order to keep space open for newer emerging truths. Here, Jung confesses,

> The journey from cloud-cuckoo-land back to reality lasted a long time. In my case Pilgrim's Progress consisted in having to climb down a thousand ladders until I could reach out my hand to the little clod of earth that I am.[26]

The practice of therapy invites ongoing expansion of the therapist's consciousness, holding capacity, and awareness of their profound limitations. In Jung's later years, says Wheelwright, he "said many times that he couldn't claim to have *the* truth, that the most he could say were that he was struggling to get to *his* truth."[27] This struggle for truth *is* what is distinctly Jungian, not an adherence to Jungian precepts. "Every psychotherapist not only has his own method—he himself is that method."[28] In the practice of therapy, as therapists and couples return again and again to the depths of their own experiences, they can use Jungian frameworks to hold that inner turning.

Because therapy starts with the known while inviting the emergence of the unknown and even the unknowable, it is both profane and sacred, mundane and miraculous. Therapists are in intimate dialogue with couples. Joseph Coppin notes that these therapeutic conversations are *erotic* dialogues, albeit sometimes quite excruciating and painful.[29] "Therapeutic eros was a name often given to compassionate empathy."[30] But each time a couple comes to therapy, therapists are reminded anew that Eros was not only the child of Aphrodite (goddess of love) but also of Ares (god of war) and that "whole love includes hatred as creativity includes destructiveness."[31] Often, this spirit of Ares, the spirit of war, is on full display when working with couples at odds with one another. The warring spirit puts tremendous pressure on the soul of a couples therapist working to help contain, normalize, contextualize, and sort through powerful and unsavory aspects of relationship.

Soul in Training

From the outset in graduate training, therapists have high expectations to become champions of change and improvement. Exposure to an array of therapeutic modalities backed with oversimplified clinical vignettes carries an implicit promise: If therapists can pull the right clinical levers at the right times, then all the tumblers will fall into place, the heavens will open, change will ensue, and everyone will live happily ever after (including the therapist). Therapists are trained to move patients *up and out* of the troubles that haunt them as quickly as possible. However, once therapists begin to practice, they encounter an altogether different clinical reality. Despite pulling all sorts of levers and paying for costly additional trainings that promise faster and greater change, intimate encounters with the actual human psyche quickly reveal the truth: *If* change can happen, it only occurs in the soul's time, not in chronologic time, despite a therapist's most heroic efforts. "Any essential change, or even a slight improvement," Jung says, "has always been a miracle."[32] While his statement insults the heroic ego, one need only look as far as the extra weight around one's midsection to realize its truth.

If heroic efforts at change are futile, then what is the so-called goal of therapy? Jung observes that the big problems in life are not so much solved as outgrown.[33] Healing, if it can occur, requires painstaking movement down, in, and toward the suffering. Outgrowing something is frustratingly circular work requiring everyone's patience as they are brought back, time and again, to the crux of the matter. A lifetime may not be enough for the psyche to fully digest its most difficult experiences. After all, ninety-year-olds *still* wonder about what happened to them when they were little.

In this light, therapists can tend the process(es) that help couples begin to *outgrow* their problems. The ability to outgrow something requires an increased capacity for the partners' psyches to hold more and more of the truth while allowing time enough to metabolize it. If you are skeptical, think back to things that took up so much time, energy, and worry, and notice that some of them now rest a little easier. Philosopher and psychologist Noel Cobb adds:

> I see psychotherapy as a work which should model itself on the crafts and should take its analogies from the arts rather than from medicine, physics or technology. No 'cure,' no 'treatment,' no 'repair' or 'adjustment of faulty functioning,' but something crafty and seaworthy, imaginative and well-fashioned, as well as aesthetic and deft.[34]

Marvin Spiegelman asked some leading Jungian analysts from around the world, many of whom Jung had either known or analyzed, to discuss their approach to therapy.[35] The title of each essay was simply *How I Do It* and it captured the essence of each therapist's approach. As a practicing therapist (Delmedico) still in search of ways to relieve my clinical anxiety, I held out hope that as I read the book, I would finally get to peek behind the curtain and learn the secret. To my dismay, each therapist's approach was unique. By describing such widely varying approaches, Spiegelman's book re-encourages therapists to deepen into their individual clinical authenticity, to honor their strengths as well as blind spots—because there will always be blind spots.

Excursion: Petty Squabbles

Therapists find that couples argue about the damnedest things. They pay hundreds and thousands of dollars to fight in front of someone else over dishwasher stacking, toilet seat position, thermostat settings, the laundry, kids' homework, who leaves the lights on, who cannot clean up after themselves, and so on. These mundane, everyday things become the de facto battle lines for couples' trench warfare. Despite all our training and so-called expertise, we remain painfully aware that this is also true in our own relationships!

When partners refuse to give an inch, relationships end over these seemingly trivial yet irreconcilable differences, the stuff no one wants to take seriously and that everyone is embarrassed to talk about.

Soul and soulful ways of working with couples begin and end right down in the muck of things. The slow, meticulous work of therapy *is* the sifting and sorting of the mess of life in search of the alchemical gold. This gold is already in a couple's possession when they arrive for treatment, albeit hidden in the mountain of seemingly insignificant matters. They often call themselves on it, confessing to the therapist, *I can't believe we keep fighting this much over such silly things.* Soul-making occurs in this ever-patient, carefully attuned listening to everything, no matter how seemingly trivial, in order to hear the fuller story. Only when everything is out on the table can it be sifted, sorted, and reconstituted. Then a couple's swords can be refashioned into plowshares. Stay down in the muck; therein lies the gold.

Soul and Care of Self

By the time couples seek therapy, they are usually in a regressed psychological state, which puts pressure on the soul of the therapist. Donald Meltzer of the Tavistock Clinic describes these couples as already "involved with one another in a very infantile way and need parental guidance.... They are not seeking investigation but are coming to be instructed, chastised, or told to love one another, and so on."[36] Therapists, out of exasperation or desperation, may find their own capacity diminished due to the overt and covert demands to be referee, judge, jury, parent, soothsayer, savior, or ally for at least one of the partners.

Holding clinical space for angry, hurting, and hurtful childlike parts of adult couples quickly returns therapists to their earliest wounding. One therapist told of wetting their pants during a couple's session early in their career when one partner suddenly became enraged. The live anger in the room immediately brought them back to their own family of origin difficulties. Other therapists report being unable to speak, think, or act while couples fight on and on. Others have thrown up after sessions. These are all calls to soul work—the therapist's need for tending their own soul. Jung says,

> The acceptance of oneself is the essence of the moral problem.... That I feed the hungry, that I forgive an insult, that I love my enemy ... all these are undoubtedly great virtues.... But what if I should discover that the least amongst them all ... that I myself stand in need of the alms of my own kindness ... what then?[37]

Jung's words echo the old adage, "The cobbler's child has the worst shoes." With the therapist's attention on serving others, they often disregard, overlook, or discount their own souls (soles).

Perhaps a therapist's best strategy for tending soul is to dedicate time to their own individual therapy. Otherwise, "we remain blind, despite everything and everybody."[38] In the past, committing to personal therapy was a primary criterion for licensure. Jung was an early and strong proponent of training analysis because he knew that "anyone who does not understand himself cannot understand others and can never be psychotherapeutically effective unless he has first treated himself with the same medicine."[39]

Soul and Death

Couples therapists are called upon to tend relationships at every conceivable stage and for a wide variety of issues. The list of stages includes couples who are dating or want pre-marital counseling, are starting a family or launching kids, or are considering separation or divorce. Issues arise from weddings, pregnancies, abortions, births, miscarriages, parenting conflicts, affairs, sex problems, old wounding, addictions, violence, subsequent marriages, blended families, rape, incest, domestic violence, permanent disabilities, terminal illnesses, and the deaths of loved ones, to name just a few. Therapists are called upon to tend soul in all of these circumstances. Even at the beginning of relationships, there are endings that demand special attention as couples grieve the loss of the honeymoon stage. "Endings," a chapter in Thomas Moore's *Soul Mates*, dares to remind the reader that all things, sooner or later, end.[40] At their most mythopoetic, couples therapists can be considered Angels of Death or *psychopomps*, charged with ferrying partners and relationships through excruciating periods of dying and death in order to allow for new ways of being to emerge.

Soul and Typology

The effect of psychological type, discussed in Chapter 4, is frequently over-looked when considering the soul of the therapist. Fundamental typological and temperamental differences among therapists and between therapists and couples can be sources of doubt and insecurity. Early surveys of Jungian therapists showed a predominance of introversion and intuition,[41] while Wheelwright believes that Freudians tend more toward extraversion and sensation.[42] However, therapists of all psychological types practice all types of therapy and are in relationships with all types of partners.

Couples therapy places typological pressures on the soul of the therapist in various ways. For example, heavily introverted therapists may find themselves exceptionally drained after couples sessions, which more heavily draw on precious extraverted resources than individual therapy. Or a strong thinking therapist may find themselves typologically exhausted after a session with a couple awash in feelings, a function they may have little personal access to. Noticing and naming this typological tiredness and taking time to be with one's Self are ways therapists tend their own souls. It may require additional quiet time alone at the end of a clinical day to rejuvenate. Also, the very nature of the work regularly draws the therapist into their unconscious and toward their inferior function in search of what may be missing in the therapy. If their inferior function erupts in session, therapists may find the experience unsettling. Regardless, all the therapist's typological functions are soulfully acted upon as they seek to attune to each partner and consider the clinical material. At the end of the workday, therapists may depart with a feeling of having come a bit undone or of being more loosely held together. In such moments, the soul is in need of care.

Soul and the Sacred

Jung once remarked that among the hundreds of people he treated worldwide, the one common denominator was a spiritual problem.[43] His patients were suffering because they had lost or outgrown their reasons for living, and none of them recovered unless they found a new reason to carry on. Some couples who enter therapy today, like Jung's patients, have discovered that the vicissitudes of relationship have a way of forcing issues of meaning and purpose to consciousness. For instance, couples who made sacred vows to one another show up for treatment suffering under their weight. Even if they have not made vows, some kind of spiritual problem usually lies at the bottom of relational discontent. Thus, therapists working soulfully are also working at the heart of spiritual problems. Little wonder that, theology and belief systems aside, many therapists consider the practice of therapy to be sacred.

Namaste, a term from the Hindu and Yogic traditions, can be translated as "The sacred in me recognizes the sacred in you."[44] With a couple's dreams of happily-ever-after shattered, they often lose sight of the sacred in each other and are usually in some form of spiritual crisis. A Jungian approach to couples therapy accounts for spiritual problems and invites an ever-deepening, more authentic, living relationship to them. With a daily approach to the *living mystery* of what is happening inside partners and between them, couples therapy can rightfully be called a spiritual practice regardless of the therapist's or the partners' religious affiliations, if any.[45]

How To Care for Soul

While it is essential for therapists to tend their own souls, guidelines for doing so are rare. What does it look like in practice? Framing a specific answer is impossible because each therapist is utterly unique, as are the demands of their ever-emerging Self. However, some skills and habits for tending the therapist's soul can be useful at two distinct times: while in sessions with couples, and outside of them.

During sessions, therapists can learn to deeply attune to their patients while simultaneously remaining attuned to themselves. The mind is extraordinarily fast, and it is very good at multitasking. Such multitasking is important because therapy, which is psychologically activating for everyone, kindles the soul of the therapist. So, as they listen to the couple's language and images, therapists can follow the flow of their own images and thoughts, noticing when they are attending to the dialog and when they become distracted—and whether that train of thought leading away may, in fact, be meaningful to the work. Though we have frequently encouraged curiosity and warm interest, therapists are ordinary people: they grow bored, sleepy, or disinterested; or their thinking shifts from clear to foggy, or they shut down, or they want to run away. Therapists can train some of their attention on themselves, noticing when they wax poetic and when they are rendered mute.

Therapists also can tend their soul in intimate clinical moments by noting somatic and emotional cues: ongoing changes in their breathing, heart rate, and bodily sensations, as well as the ebbs and flows of fear, anxiety, happiness, elation, giddiness, joy, sadness, anger, rage, and disgust. They can be attentive to acute shifts in mood and track how their own archetypal energies roil and undulate. Aside from the clinical usefulness of countertransference responses, any and all of this information may well reveal a need in the therapist's soul.

Since so much of soul work is expressed in images, therapists can tend their own soul in session by observing their fantasies and reveries moment by moment. Such fantasies may have clinical relevance as suggested above, or speak to the state of their own soul, or both. When therapists honor their own inner images, figures, and metaphors as they arise and recede in session, they are tending their own soul. This does not come at the expense of the couple; empathic attunement expands to include everyone, the couple and the therapist, with the result that more clinical space becomes available in the room, not less. All are cared for, in real time, together—dissolving the unnatural either/or dichotomy that splits the healer from the wounded.

Outside of sessions, therapists tend their own soul by taking time to re-regulate themselves through known or familiar practices that restore the nervous system to a calm state. (The Japanese speak of restoring one's *wa*, a short word that means harmony with all things.) They can process unmetabolized clinical material via reverie, journaling, peer consultation, or supervision, especially if the work has touched old painful wounds. When working with couples has generated personal insights, therapists might take time to revisit their own relational wounds to integrate what they learned. Since couples therapy brings us to our deepest wounding, therapists might also want to consider additional therapy as care of their soul.

Therapists can also tend soul by cultivating a full life outside the confines of professional practice, far from the gestalt of wounds, healing, therapy, and psychological insight. Follow the heart to discover activities and people that replenish your vitality and set aside enough time for them. Honor your soul's unique calling—which can be anything—without explanation, rationalization, or defense. Dance, yoga, journaling, poetry, pottery, fencing, gardening, stonework, book club, trivia night, gaming, dreamwork, comedy, writing, exercise, cooking; the list is endless. The only requirement is soulful interest. Period. (And probably a measure of joy.) Doing something in an attempt to be well-rounded is an ego move, and only turns the activity into yet another chore in life.

In tending our own souls, interest wells up from deep within. At first, it may only be a faint whisper. *Wait, wood ducks? Do I really want to try and learn how to carve wood ducks?*

Imagine that.

Conclusion

As therapists continually refine their practice, moving toward greater knowledge, skill, and depth, they discover the depths in their own souls. It cannot be otherwise. Traveling the labyrinthine ways of psyche is a lifelong journey. Even as you become adept at following its mysteries, you are always the student, never the master. In the end, a Jungian approach to couples therapy does not emulate Jung. Instead, you craft something authentic and individual, doing the work only you can do and perhaps "laying an infinitesimal grain in the scales of humanity's soul. Small and invisible as this contribution may be, it is yet an *opus magnum*."[46]

Notes

1 Raimy 1950, p. 93.
2 Bush 2015.
3 Rowan & Jacobs 2002.

4 Guggenbühl-Craig 1971.
5 Remen 1997, p. 178.
6 Jung 1935, para. 319.
7 Freud 1910.
8 Jung 1931, para. 163.
9 Sedgwick 2001, pp. 137–138.
10 Cambray 2009.
11 Jung 1946a, para. 179.
12 Tresan 1996.
13 Hillman 1965, p. 132.
14 Jung 1923, p. 10.
15 Jung 1973, p. 456.
16 Bion 1967.
17 Wolf 2005, p. 1.
18 From "The Road Not Taken" (Frost 2016, p. 133, line 13).
19 Jung 1946b, para. 365.
20 Sedgwick 2001, pp. 48–49.
21 Sedgwick 2001.
22 Sedgwick 2001, p. 48.
23 Wheelwright 1982, p. 59.
24 Hannah 1976, p. 78.
25 Campbell 1991, p. 15.
26 Jung 1973, p. 19.
27 Wheelwright 1982, p. 98.
28 Jung 1945, para. 198.
29 Coppin 1996.
30 Hillman 1972, p. 87.
31 Hillman 1972, p. 88.
32 Jung 1934, para. 815.
33 Jung 1957, p. 15.
34 Cobb 1992, p. 25.
35 Spiegelman 1988.
36 Fisher & Meltzer 1995, p. 119.
37 Jung 1932, para. 520.
38 Jung 1946b, para. 449.
39 Jung 1973, p. 456.
40 Moore 1994.
41 Bradway & Wheelwright 1978.
42 Wheelwright 1982.
43 Jung 1932.
44 Oxhandler 2017, p. 168.
45 See Corbett 1996, 2011; Epstein 1995, 2007.
46 Jung 1946b, para. 449.

References

Bion, W. (1967). Notes on memory and desire. *The Psychoanalytic Forum*, 2(3), 271–280.
Bradway, K., & Wheelwright, J. (1978) The psychological type of the analyst. *Journal of Analytical Psychology*, 23(3), 211–225. https://doi.org/10.1111/j.1465-5922.1978.00211.x.
Bush, A. D. (2015). *Simple self-care for therapists*. W. W. Norton & Company.

Cambray, J. (2009). *Synchronicity.* Texas A&M University Press.

Campbell, J. (1991). *Reflections on the art of living.* (D. K. Obson, Ed.). Harper Perennial.

Cobb, N. (1992). *Archetypal imagination.* Lindisfarne Press.

Coppin, J. (1996). *Erotic dialogues.* (Doctoral dissertation). Retrieved from ProQuest Dissertations and Theses database. (UMI No. LD03615)

Corbett, L. (1996). *The religious function of the psyche.* Routledge.

Corbett, L. (2011). *The sacred cauldron.* Chiron.

Epstein, M. (1995). *Thoughts without a thinker.* Basic Books.

Epstein, M.(2007). *Psychotherapy without the self.* Yale University Press.

Fisher, J. & Meltzer, D. (1995). Donald Meltzer in discussion. In S. Ruszczynski & J. V. Fisher (Eds.), *Intrusiveness and intimacy in the couple* (pp. 107–144). Karnac.

Freud, S. (1910). 'Wild' psycho-analysis. *SE* XI.

Frost, R. (2016). *The Collected Poems of Robert Frost.* Chartwell Books.

Guggenbühl-Craig, A. (1971). *Power in the helping professions.* Spring Publications.

Hannah, B. (1976). *Jung: His life and work.* Putnam.

Hillman, J. (1965). *Suicide and the soul* (2nd ed.). Spring Publications.

Hillman, J. (1972). *The myth of analysis.* Northwestern University Press.

Jung, C. G. (1923). *The integration of the personality.* Routledge & Kegan Paul.

Jung, C. G. (1931). Problems of modern psychotherapy. *CW* 16.

Jung, C. G. (1932). Psychotherapists or the clergy. *CW* 11.

Jung, C. G. (1934). The soul and death. *CW* 8.

Jung, C. G. (1935). *The Tavistock lectures. CW18.*

Jung, C. G. (1945). Medicine and psychotherapy. *CW16.*

Jung, C. G. (1946a). Psychotherapy and a philosophy of life. *CW* 16.

Jung, C. G. (1946b). The psychology of the transference. *CW* 16.

Jung, C. G. (1957). Commentary on "The secret of the golden flower."*CW* 13.

Jung, C. G. (1973). *C. G. Jung: Letters,* Vol. 1 (G. Adler & A. Jaffé, Eds.) (R. F. C. Hull, Trans.). Routledge & Kegan Paul.

Moore, T. (1994). *Soul Mates.* Harper Perennial.

Oxhandler, H. (2017). Namaste theory. *Religions,* 8(9), 168–179. https://doi.org/10.3390/rel8090168.

Raimy, V. A. (1950). *Training in clinical psychology.* Prentice Hall.

Remen, R. N. (1997). *Kitchen table wisdom.* Riverhead Books.

Rowan, J., & Jacobs, M. (2002). *The therapist's use of self.* Open University Press.

Sedgwick, D. (2001). *Introduction to Jungian psychotherapy.* Routledge.

Spiegelman, J. M. (1988). *Jungian analysts.* Falcon Press.

Tresan, D. I. (1996). Jungian metapsychology and neurobiological theory. *Journal of Analytical Psychology,* 41, 399–436.

Wheelwright, J. B. (1982). *Saint George and the dandelion.* C. G. Jung Institute of San Francisco.

Wolf, F. A. (2005). *Dr. Quantum's little book of big ideas.* Moment Point.

Index

Note: bold page numbers indicate tables; italic page numbers indicate figures; page numbers followed by n refer to notes.

For Product Safety Concerns and Information please contact our EU
representative GPSR@taylorandfrancis.com
Taylor & Francis Verlag GmbH, Kaufingerstraße 24, 80331 München, Germany

www.ingramcontent.com/pod-product-compliance
Lightning Source LLC
Chambersburg PA
CBHW070343270326
41926CB00017B/3960

9 78 10 3 2 68 7 98 8